Oduntan holds a B.Sc. (Hons) in Optometry from the University of Benin, Nigeria and a Ph.D. from The City University, London, UK. He has over thirty years teaching experience in low vision care from various Departments of Optometry, including King Saud University, Saudi Arabia, University of Limpopo, South Africa, University of KwaZulu-Natal, Durban, South Africa. He currently teaches low vision care at Madonna University, Nigeria. He has published widely in high impact Ophthalmology, Ophthalmic Sciences, Anatomy and Optometry Journals. He has published a monograph on visual impairment and a chapter on mental health and psychology in Africa.

This book is dedicated to forerunners
of low vision care and education.

Oduntan

CONTEMPORARY LOW VISION CARE

AUSTIN MACAULEY PUBLISHERS™
LONDON · CAMBRIDGE · NEW YORK · SHARJAH

Copyright © Oduntan 2024

The right of Oduntan to be identified as author of this work has been asserted by the author in accordance with sections 77 and 78 of the Copyright, Designs and Patents Act 1988.

All rights reserved. No part of this publication may be reproduced, stored in a retrieval system, or transmitted in any form or by any means, electronic, mechanical, photocopying, recording, or otherwise, without the prior permission of the publishers.

Any person who commits any unauthorized act in relation to this publication may be liable to criminal prosecution and civil claims for damages.

The medical information in this book is not advice and should not be treated as such. Do not substitute this information for the medical advice of physicians. The information is general and intended to better inform readers of their health care. Always consult your doctor for your individual needs.

A CIP catalogue record for this title is available from the British Library.

ISBN 9781528990202 (Paperback)
ISBN 9781528990219 (ePub-e-book)

www.austinmacauley.com

First Published 2024
Austin Macauley Publishers Ltd®
1 Canada Square
Canary Wharf
London
E14 5AA

This book was written during my time working at the University of Limpopo, Tufloop Campus and University of KwaZulu-Natal, Westville Campus, Durban, South Africa. Therefore, I would like to thank the management of those institutions for providing the resources that facilitated the writing and completion of the book. I also wish to thank my previous students at King Saud University, Saudi Arabia; University of Limpopo and University of KwaZulu-Natal for the experience I gained while teaching them low vision care.

Many individuals contributed in one way or another during the preparation of this book. I would like to thank them all. I am particularly grateful to Ms Sanchia Jogessar and Mr. Danhauser for demonstrating the use of low vision devices in this book. I am greatly indebted to Mr. Steenkamp of the University of Limpopo, who drew the figures and Mr. Robert Sandrock, University of Limpopo who prepared the photographs of devices shown in this book. Also, I wish to thank Mrs. Hazel Sacharowitz of the University of Johannesburg and Dr. Emeka Uzor, Madonna University, Nigeria, for their useful criticism of the draft of the book. My gratitude also goes to the editors, African Vision and Eye Health (formally The South African Optometrist) and author of all journals consulted in writing this book.

Table of Contents

Synopsis	11
Preface	13
Chapter 1: Definitions of Visual Impairment and Related Terms	14
References	26
Bibliography	28
Chapter 2: Impacts of Visual Impairment and Rehabilitation of the Visually Impaired	29
References	49
Bibliography	51
Chapter 3: Clinical Assessment of Adult Low Vision Patients	54
References	82
Bibliography	83
Chapter 4: Clinical Assessment of Children With Low Vision	84
References	93
Bibliography	94
Chapter 5: Principles of Magnification in Low Vision Care	95
References	109
Bibliography	110
Chapter 6: Prescribing Assistive Devices for Low Vision Patients	111
References	128
Bibliography	130

Chapter 7: Optical Assistive Devices for Low Vision Patients   131

References   166

Bibliography   169

Chapter 8: Non-Optical Assistive Devices for Low Vision Patients   170

References   190

Bibliography   191

Chapter 9: Visual Field Enhancement for Low Vision Patients   192

References   197

Chapter 10: Incorporating Low Vision Care Into an Eye Care Practice   199

Bibliography   205

Synopsis

Low vision is a condition in which, a person has poor vision due to certain visual disorders, and the vision cannot be improved to normal level by medical, surgical or optical means. The visual disorders can be oculo-visual in nature, such as glaucoma; possibly due to ocular manifestations of systemic diseases such as diabetes or may be due to other visual disturbances. Consequences of low vision may include the inability to see clearly at near or far distances, or the inability to see objects in the peripheral aspects of the visual field. This visual condition can lead to inability to perform activities of daily living which may include the inability to read normal sized prints at a near distance or the inability to see distant objects such as recognising people faces. This vision status may lead to psychological problems such as feelings of insecurity, low self-concept, anxiety or depression. It can also result in poor quality of life.

Although, low vision cannot be improved to a 'normal level', people with such visual conditions can be assisted to perform certain limited activities after appropriate visual rehabilitation, which may include provision of optical, non-optical or electronic visual devices and or appropriate non-visual devices. Occasionally, if there are indications that the patient exhibits psychological manifestations, rehabilitation may include psychological management. The person with the condition should be seen as a whole person with several social, economic, spiritual and psychological needs. Attempts should be made to find solutions to all the patient's needs during rehabilitation program.

Eye care practitioners, who have received specialized training in low vision care are usually the coordinators of these types of rehabilitation programs. Their role is usually to use magnification, minification, electronic methods and other appropriate methods to enhance task performance, such as reading at near or distance for the patient. Also, they may provide non-optical devices to provide comfort for the patient while reading. Further, they may need to refer the patient to other professionals for necessary non-visual management such as counselling before the visual needs are attended to or they may refer the client to other professionals such as orientation and mobility instructors, after the visual aspects of the rehabilitation have been attended to.

This low vision care book explains what low vision is, the possible causes and its consequences. Methods of visual rehabilitation including, eye and visual examination, calculation of magnification required by the patient to perform specific tasks, provision of optical, non-optical and electronic assistive devices and follow-up care are described in the book. The last chapter of the book is devoted to advice on how eye care practitioners can incorporate low vision care into their existing eye care practices. This book will be useful to eye care practitioners and other professionals such as Occupational therapists, Social workers and Orientation & mobility instructors who are interested in, or who wish to develop an interest in low vision care.

Oduntan

Preface

Low vision is a major health problem worldwide, impacting seriously on everyday lives of those affected. It affects a larger population worldwide than blindness. Functionally, low vision can be defined as visual acuity or visual field loss, which after medical and or regular optical intervention still results in the individual not being able to perform visually guided tasks as those with normal vision perform. This definition highlights the fact that following the best eye care intervention by professionals (Ophthalmologists and or Optometrists), an individual with low vision cannot perform most tasks that normal sighted individual can perform. However, following further visual assessment and provision of low vision devices, such individuals can perform certain specific tasks. Visual aspect of low vision care is a specialty area of eye care, however, total rehabilitation of those with the condition often require a multidisciplinary approach, involving both the eye care practitioners and other health care professionals. The assistance of professionals such as psychologists, counsellors and occupational therapists in order to provide a comprehensive service to the patient. This eye care and other professional intervention, referred to as 'comprehensive interdisciplinary rehabilitation', enables a person with low vision to live relatively productive, enjoyable and fulfilling life.

This book was written to provide an introductory information to eye care practitioners and other health care professionals who may wish to gain an insight into low vision care. It provides information relating to the various definitions of low vision, causes and prevalence of low vision worldwide, with emphasis on aspects of low vision patient rehabilitation. Although the book is introductory in nature, it provides a significant information necessary for low vision rehabilitation. The book will also be useful to all health care professionals who have interest in low vision care.

Oduntan

Chapter 1
Definitions of Visual Impairment and Related Terms

Low vision and blindness constitute visual impairment. Visual impairment can simply be defined as reduction in visual function/s of a person, ranging from low vision to total blindness. It could be expressed in terms of reduction in visual acuity, visual field or contrast sensitivity of a person. Therefore, visual impairment can be quantified in terms of visual acuity or visual, field, but infrequently as contrast sensitivity loss. Traditionally, visual impairment is classified based on best corrected vision (Best corrected visual acuity) in the better eye. In the past, World Health Organization[1] defined low vision as visual acuity ranging from worse than 6/18 (3/10) (20/70) (0.3) to better than 3/60 (1/20) (20/400) (0.05). Acuity worse than this may constitute blindness. Blindness was defined as acuity reduction ranging from 3/60 (1/20) (20/400) (0.05) to counting finger (CF) at 1 meter (1/50) (1/50) (6/300) (20/1200) (0.02). Visual field loss less than 20 degrees but better than 10 degrees around the central fixation point in the better eye, with best correction also constitutes low vision. Blindness is defined as visual field loss ranging from 10° to no light perception[1].

In the current WHO[2] definitions, however, visual impairment is defined or classified based on presenting visual acuity and best corrected visual acuity. Low vision is defined as presenting visual acuity from worse than 6/18 (3/10) (20/70) (0.3) to better than 3/60 (1/20) (20/400) (0.05), with current correction, if any. Blindness is defined as visual better than 3/60, (1/20), (20/400), (0.05 logMAR) to light perception. Visual field less than 10° in the better eye constitutes blindness. Classification based on presenting visual acuity allows those conditions that are due to correctable anomalies such as refractive errors to be recognized as visual impairment as well[3]. Many authors including the author of this book still prefer those old definitions, because they are of the opinion that low vision should be diagnosed after thorough refraction and correction.

Following optical correction and or other forms of eye care intervention, if the vision cannot be improved to normal level of vision, the person is considered to have uncorrectable visual impairment. Impaired vision, whether due correctable or uncorrectable disorder, is frequently associated with visual disability and poor task performance. It is, however, important to note the importance of monocular and binocular visual impairment, because loss of vision in only one eye is obviously of less disability than binocular impairment. There are many people with one eye, who perform jobs just as efficiently as normally sighted ones. However, monocular disability may cause serious visual disability in certain functions and may result in inability of the person involved to partake in certain physical, economic and social activities.

Visual impairment can be classified on the basis of difficulty in task performance. However, this should only be done after appropriate medical intervention and or thorough refraction has been done to improve the visual acuity of the person to the normal value or otherwise. A patient with active ocular or systemic disease may have poor vision that affects visual performance, but following appropriate and successful ophthalmological or surgical management, he or she may have normal vision restored. A person with uncorrected -10.00 diopters of myopia may only be able to read 6/60 acuity letter but following proper ophthalmic correction, he or she may be able to read 6/6 or even smaller acuity letters. Also, it should be noted that a person may be able to read 6/6 or 6/5 Snellen acuity letters at far and near, however, if he or she has visual field less than 30 degrees in the eye with greater visual field, he or she may still be classified as a low vision person. This is because the reduced field may not enable him to perform optimally in many vocational, avocational, social, and daily living activities or tasks.

Traditionally, and in the real sense of it, vision loss that cannot be managed medically, surgically or optically to achieve normal level of vision that permits the person to perform activities of daily living without the use of devices known as low vision devices is termed low vision. As mentioned above, WHO[2] has classified visual impairment (low vision and blindness) based on corrected and uncorrected (presenting) vision. In the context of this book, low vision refers to the visual impairment that is not correctable by medical and or optical means, thereby requiring special adaptive devices to perform visually guided tasks.

Low vision is commonly known as partial sight. Low vision and blindness can result from several disorders which include congenital anomalies (such as albinism or congenital cataract) or can be a consequence of acquired eye diseases (such as eye injury, eye diseases, or other eye conditions). Many people with low vision experience difficulties with activities such reading, watching television, walking around, as well as engaging in several other daily living activities such as cooking, shopping and self-keeping. There are, however, a wide variety of assistive devices and environmental modifications that can enable a low vision patient see better in order to perform certain limited visual tasks.

Definitions and classifications of low vision and blindness are important because of the socio-economic status that associated with them. Many visually impaired individuals depend on grant from the government to meet their financial needs. Also, qualification to partake in certain local, national and international sporting activities or competitions meant for the visually impaired require potential participants to be examined visually and their visual status indicated. Therefore, they need to be examined and classified as having low vision or blindness based on existing definitions or classifications before they can access such grants or other economic activities or partake in certain sporting competitions. Visually impaired children need to be classified as having low vision or blindness in order to be admitted into schools for the visually impaired.

Definitions and Classifications of Low Vision

There are many definitions of low vision in the literature and new ones emerge from time to time. This is due to many factors such as the differences in the criteria used in the definitions. Some definitions are based on impairment of measurable visual functions such as visual acuity, contrast sensitivity or visual field, while others are based on functional consequences of low vision or blindness (disability or handicap). Even, when the same visual function such as visual acuity is used to define low vision or blindness, there may be value variations as one author may use 6/18 as the cut off point for normality, whereas another may use a different value such as 6/12. Such differences are based on the experience or perception of different practitioners on what acuity levels that are needed to perform certain task.

Also, while some definitions are based on visual acuity or visual field values independently, both functions need to be used when certain functions need to be performed therefore both functions are used in the definition of low vision by some authors. Further, in some definitions, the visual acuity and visual field values are varied in the definitions depending on the degree of visual field loss, and vice versa. Therefore, the better the visual field value, the poorer the visual acuity used to indicate visual impairment. Further, another important reason why there are differences in the definitions of low vision or blindness definitions is the fact that different countries adopt different values for the definitions. This is partly because different countries use different values of visual functions to determine who qualifies for state grants and other state benefits.

In view of the different reasons stated above, different definitions of low vision and blindness will be found in the textbooks. In view of the several visual parameters and functional consequences that may be involved in visual impairment, it is difficult to define low vision or blindness in one sentence.

In this book, low vision is defined as bilateral reduced visual acuity or visual field restriction which is severe enough to interfere with daily living activities performance and vision cannot be improved by medical, regular ophthalmic or contact lenses intervention, but requires low vision devices and or environmental modifications for performance improvement. The visual acuity values of worse than 6/18 but better than 3/60 (6/120) and central visual field of 10° or better but less than 30° are assumed for this definition. Worse acuity values and less visual field values are considered to be blindness.

The most commonly used visual functions in the definitions of low vision are visual acuity and visual field. Also, contrast sensitivity values are occasionally used to define low vision because it has disabling capacity in daily activities performance, just as the visual acuity and visual field loss. Existing definitions of low vision that could be found in the literature include the following:

i. Corrected visual acuity less than 6/18 (20/60) or a visual field less than 30 degrees[4]
ii. Inability to read a newspaper at a normal reading distance of 40 centimeters with the best refractive correction[5]

iii. Reduced central visual acuity or visual field loss, which even with the best optical correction provided by regular lenses, still results in visual impairment from performance standpoint. This definition assumes that the visual loss is bilateral, that some form of vision remains, and that regular lenses do not include additions greater than +4.00 diopters or low vision devices[6]. The regular lenses according to the author of this definition include contact lenses and intra-ocular lenses. Although, regular lenses may not improve vision, this does not mean that a patient cannot benefit from the use of optical devices referred to as low vision optical devices. Therefore, the use of such devices are excluded from this definition. This definition is also tied to a reduced level of visual performance, which means that a certain level of disability must accompany the visual impairment and the visual disability must be of such a magnitude that it adversely affects visual task performance.

iv. Vision in the better eye between 6/18 (20/60) and 3/60 (20/400) with the best refractive correction or visual field less than 30 degrees. This definition implies that if a patient has visual acuity worse than 3/60 (6/120) (20/400), he or she is no longer a low vision patient, but is blind[1]

v. It has been advised that classifying children as having low vision should be done with caution. Only children having a fully developed visual system can be classified with certainty and not infants and young children. This is because the developmental influence of vision during early life is so potent that even very rudimentary residual vision may be capable of developing and promoting general visual development to some extent later in life[7]

vi. Visual impairment sufficient to cause a disability (visual acuity of <6/12)[8].

vii. Defective vision of a substantially and permanently handicapping nature caused by congenital defect, illness or injury. This was tied with visual acuity values between 3/60 and 6/60 when the visual field is full. The visual acuity should be 6/24 when the visual field is moderately constricted, or 6/18 or better, when the visual field is grossly reduced[9].

viii. This definition emphasizes the adverse functional consequences of reduced visual field in the presence of fairly good central visual acuity.

ix. Disabling visual impairment, which cannot be corrected medically, surgically or with conventional eye glasses[10,11].
x. A condition of reduced visual acuity that, even with the best refractive correction, results in impaired visual performance[12].
xi. An impairment of vision preventing a person from satisfactorily performing visual tasks with a conventional optical correction[13].

It will be observed that many of the above definitions refer to best corrected visual acuity. This is important as those with correctable visual disorders can be assisted with appropriate refractive management for them to acquire normal vision. Many low vision definitions directly or indirectly refer to inability to function optimally in everyday activities because of visual impairment or disability. Visual field loss adversely affects task performance such as reading or walking. Location of the field defect as well as the location of the residual visual field are important because a centrally located 20 degrees visual field generally affords better visual capacity compared to a peripherally located 20 degrees field.

Occasionally, an eye care practitioner is approached to assist in classifying low vision patients for one reason or another, which may include qualification for a disability grant or taking part in sports. In deciding whether a patient is a low vision or blind patient, one needs to evaluate both the person's visual acuity and visual field. Consider the following cases to appreciate the importance of this statement:

Example 1

A 45 years old diabetic retinopathy patient came for classification. The best corrected visual acuities at distance and near were as follows:

Uncorrected visual acuity Corrected visual acuity
Right eye (OD) 6/30 6/25
Left eye (OS) 6/30 6/25
Both eyes (OU) 6/25 6/20
Visual field: OD 120°, OS 120°

On the basis of the current visual acuity alone, one can conclude that this patient is a low vision patient and assume that unless a low vision aid is provided for him or her, he or she may have difficulty performing daily activities such as reading newspaper or seeing writing on the chalkboard.

Example 2

A 25 years old lady came to your clinic with history of *retinitis pigmentosa*. The visual acuities were as follows:

Uncorrected visual acuity Corrected visual acuity

Righteye (OD) 6/7.5 6/6

Left eye (OS) 6/6 6/6

Both eyes (OU) 6/6 6/6

Central field around the fixation point:

OD 10°

OS 15°

On the basis of visual acuity alone, one may conclude that this patient is not a low vision patient. In spite of the good visual acuity, however, due to the field restriction, this patient definitely has low vision. Therefore, visual acuity or visual field alone should not be used to decide that a patient has low vision or not.

Blindness

World Health Organization (WHO)[14] defined blindness as inability to perform tasks, which normally require gross vision, without relying on other senses. Blindness is often defined as visual acuity worse than 3/60 or visual field less than 10 degrees around the fixation point[15]. Also, blindness is often classified as functional blindness or legal blindness as defined below.

Functional blindness has been defined as severely reduced visual acuity or visual field loss that cannot be improved by medical or surgical, optical or any other intervention methods, to a level that can allow a person to perform visual tasks at all or without difficulty.

Legal Blindness

Like low vision, there are many definitions for legal blindness, which include inability to perform any work for which visual acuity is essential and is tied to visual acuity of 3/60 (20/400). Also, legal blindness has been defined as corrected visual acuity of 20/200 (6/60) or worse, or visual field of 20 degrees or less in any meridian in the better eye[16].

Further, legal blindness has been classified as a significantly restricted visual field irrespective of how good the visual acuity is. It has also been defined as visual acuity of 6/60 (20/200) or less, or visual field of 20 degrees or less in the better eye[1].

Monocular Blindness

Monocular blindness refers to visual acuity less than 3/60 or visual field less than 10 degrees in one eye, while there is normal vision in the other. Monocular blindness can occur as a result of many conditions including trauma, cataract, retinal detachment, and optic nerve lesion. It is essential to note that monocular blindness has very little functional significance if the other eye is free of disease and has normal visual acuity and relatively extensive or full visual field. Many functions or tasks can be performed monocularly, except those that require binocular stereopsis. Even in those cases, the person can employ monocular cues to do the work to a certain extent. A monocular person, however, can be barred from engaging in certain jobs requiring active binocularity, if he or she would constitute a danger to himself, herself or others. A person with one eye may not be recommended to be an aeroplane pilot.

Other Relevant Definitions

Visual Impairment, Visual Disorder, Visual Disability and Visual Handicap

Basic definitions of terms relating to vision loss such as visual disorder, visual impairment, visual disability and visual handicap help in understanding concept of the visual loss its etiological, structural, physiological, social and psychological ramifications. Quite often, these terms are erroneously used interchangeably as if they are synonymous. Presumably, this is because of their relationships, but indeed, each describes different aspects of vision loss. Leat et al.[8] have defined the terms as they relate to the eye and vision. In general, visual disorder relates to anatomical or physiology anomaly of the eye and/ or visual system that results in one or more abnormalities in the eye and or the visual system. Visual impairment results from visual disorder and visual disability is a consequence of visual impairment and in certain cases; visual disability may result in visual handicap. Visual disorder, visual impairment, visual disability and visual handicap therefore, are related but different terms. They are related in the sense that one can, but not necessarily lead to another. A disorder or anomaly in the eye may or may not lead to visual impairment, and the latter may exist without resulting in visual disability. Also, a visual disability may exist with or without visual handicap. These definitions are presented and commented upon below.

Visual Disorder

This refers to any deviation from the normal structure or physiology of the eye or visual system or any physiological or pathological anomaly of the eye or visual pathway.

The visual processes involve both the optical system (eye and related structures) and perceptual system (the visual pathway and relevant neural connections). Visual disorder, therefore, emanates from abnormality or structural changes or anomaly resulting from congenital or acquired structural anomaly, injury or diseases in the eye or visual pathway. In essence, a visual disorder can either be a genetic or acquired condition in the eye or visual pathway. An opacity in the crystalline lens of the eye, called cataract, is a lenticular disorder. A person can be born with such opacity or it may be acquired as a result of trauma, environmental radiations or as part of the normal aging process. The opacity can lead to visual impairment depending on its size, density and location relative to the visual axis. Also, depending on the magnitude of the impairment, it may lead to visual disability and possibly visual handicap.

Foveal hypoplasia, often associated with absence or reduced pigmentation of the uvea or the retinal pigment epithelium, as in the case of albinism can adversely affect vision depending on the degree of hypoplasia and reduction of pigmentation. Also, macular hole and macular degeneration are examples of disorders in the macular and foveal regions with a capacity to result in visual impairment. Similarly, a significant disorder in the visual pathway such as in the optic nerve, optic chiasma, optic radiation, lateral geniculate body, optic radiation or visual cortex can lead to visual impairment if both eyes are significantly affected. Subsequently, visual disability or visual handicap might ensue depending on the magnitude of the lesion.

Visual Impairment

Visual impairment is defined as a measurable loss or departure of functional capability relative to the normal variation in healthy eyes. It is a psychophysical measurement in vision, which is outside the normal range.

Visual impairment relates to quantifiable functional changes in the eyes such as visual acuity, visual field and contrast sensitivity. A disorder in the eye or other visual structures may lead to visual impairment, but not all disorders lead to visual impairment. A centrally located dense bilateral corneal or lenticular opacity may lead to visual impairment if it infringes on a significant area of the pupil, whereas, if the same opacity is peripherally located with little or no bearing on the papillary region, it will not lead to any measurable decrease in visual acuity, visual field or contrast sensitivity loss. Hence, it will not result in visual impairment. Similarly, while a centrally located 20° retinal lesion or disorder may result in significant reduction in visual acuity and contrast sensitivity and visual field, a similar magnitude of disorder located peripherally may not cause the same reduction in visual function. It should be noted, however, that a severe peripheral field loss can cause severe navigation problems for a patient.

Certain disorders, may result in visual impairment in one person but not in another. For instance, lack of pigmentation, depending on the degree in the normally pigmented structures of the eyes and foveal hypoplasia in individuals with albinism, are structural disorders that lead to visual impairment in these people. The visual involvement may include reduced visual acuity and poor contrast sensitivity in many individuals, but there are a few individuals who have albinism, having iridic hypopigmentation and foveal hypoplasia, but without visual impairment (acuity 6/18 or better). This may be related to lesser degree of hypopigmentation of the relevant ocular structures and foveal hypoplasia.

All the examples cited above imply that factors such as magnitude and location of a disorder are important in determining whether or not they will result in visual impairment. An important point to note is that visual impairment is independent on a patient's vocational and avocational engagements, hence, a patient's visual acuity or visual field value is not dependent on what he or she wants to perform visually.

Visual Disability

This refers to loss of capacity to perform a certain task as a result of visual impairment. It is any diminished or absent ability to perform a task, because of visual impairment, or lack of ability to perform a task involving vision that is needed to maintain one's desired lifestyle.

From the definition above, it is clear that visual disability refers to reduced ability or lack of capacity to perform a visually guided task. Visual disability is a consequence of visual impairment, therefore relates to reduced capacity or reduced functional ability of a person to perform activities for which vision is needed. Visual impairment may have a great impact on a person's ability to perform activities of daily living, thus resulting in visual disability. In addition, some people with certain level of visual impairment may be able to perform certain activities, but not others. For example, a person may not be able to read newspapers, house numbers or bus numbers from normal distances because of reduced visual acuity. However, he or she may, on the basis of the inability to perform these activities, be referred to as being visually disabled. The same person may, however, be able to move around freely without any assistance. On the basis of orientation and mobility difficulty, the same person is thus not visually disabled. Visual disability may, therefore be activity specific, although a visual impairment may affect several capacities.

A person with significantly reduced peripheral visual field (tunnel vision) may be able to read small print at near, but may not be able to drive a car safely because he or she will not be able to see objects that are outside his or her central field. These examples show that although visual impairment is independent of vocational and avocational tasks, visual disability is task specific. It is important to note that not all visual impairments result in visual disability. If a visual impairment is not significant to interfere with task performance, it may exist without causing a disability. Also, the degree of disability caused will differ for different tasks to be performed.

Visual Handicap

This refers to actual or perceived social, economic or psychological disadvantage, which results from a disability.

Visual handicap is a consequence of visual disability and is often associated with the degrees of physical, economic and social independence that a person experiences as a consequence of visual disability. It can be regarded as a classification of circumstances that place an individual in a disadvantaged circumstance, relative to his or her peers, when viewed from the norms of the society. A visually handicapped person often lacks privacy and independence as he or she or she may have to depend on a sighted friend or member of the family to read mails, even when such mail is personal or confidential. That dependence is a form of handicap.

A visually impaired person may be able to drive and has money to buy a car. However, he or she will not be granted a driver's license. Therefore she cannot driver himself or herself. That inability to get a driver's license is a form of handicap. A person with low vision may wish to attend social functions. The psychological factors such as fear of bumping into people or objects may prevent him or her from attending such social functions. Even if he or she manages to attend a special social function, he or she may not be able to freely relate to others as the normally sighted individuals because of inability to recognize people's faces. Visual disability may lead to difficulty in performing effectively on a job, which may eventually lead to job loss. When the latter occurs, the person may face economic difficulties. He or she may even have to depend on others for economic support, hence may become economically dependent. These dependence, exclusion, and psychological factors such as fear or poor self-concept as well as community discrimination are examples of visual handicap.

It should also be noted, however, that not all visual disabilities lead to handicap and what constitutes handicap for one person may not be for another. Determining factors may include the degree of the disability and attitude of the person. Stereotypical perception of people around the visually disabled persons may also put a person in a disadvantageous situations. Generally, there is an unfortunate perception that visually disabled persons may not perform jobs as efficiently as their normally sighted counterparts. This perception may not allow the visually disabled person to get a job easily. This perception is not always true because in certain jobs, the visually disabled person can perform just as efficiently as his or her normally sighted individuals.

References

World Health Organization. Methods of assessment of avoidable blindness. WHO offset publications. 1980; 54: 1-42.

World Health Organization (WHO). Visual disturbances and blindness. (H53-H54). http://icd.who.int/browse10/2016/ent# (Accessed 11 January, 2018).

Ryan B. Low vision. Part one - terminology and incidence. Optician. 1998; 215: 14-18.

Genensky SM. Functional classification system of visually impaired to replace the legal classification of blindness. Ann Ophthalmol. 1971; 3: 150-154.

5. Legge G. E. Three perspectives on low vision reading. Optom Vis Sci. 1991; 68: 763-769.

6. Mehr EB, Freid AN. Low vision care. Chicago: Professional Press, 1975.

7. Lindstedt E. Definition of visual impairment and their consequences in infants and small children. In: Documenta Ophthalmologica proceedings series 45: Detection and measurement of visual impairment in pre-verbal children. Jay B, ed. Boston: Martinus Nijhoff/Dr W. Junk Publishers, 1986.

8. Leat SJ, Legge GE and Bullimore MA. What is low vision? A re-definition of Definitions. Optom Vis Sci. 1999; 76: 198-221.

9. Bier N. BD8 Form. Her Majesty Office, Correction of subnormal vision. London, Butterworths. 1970.

10. Tielsch JM, Sommer A, Witt K, Katz J, Royall RM and the Baltimore eye Research Group. Blind and visual Impairment in an American urban population: the Baltimore eye survey. Arch Ophthalmol. 1990; 108: 286-290.

11. Nelson KA, Dimitrova E. Severe visual impairment in the United States and in each state. J Vis Impair & Blind. 1990; 87: 80-85.

12. Dickinson C. A step by step guide to low vision practice. Optician. 1993; 206: 26-33.

Bailey IL. A profile of low vision population. Optom monthly 1978; Feb. 137-145.

World Health Organization. Study group on the prevention of blindness. World Health Organization technical report series. Geneva; World Health Organization. 1972; 518.

Murdoch I. E., Jones BR, Cousens S, Liman I, Babalola OE, Dauda J. and Abiose A. Visual field constriction as a cause of blindness and visual impairment. Bull WHO 1997; 75:141-146.

Kirchner C. Data on blindness and visual impairment in the USA. Resource manual on social demographic characteristics, education, employment, income and services delivery. New York: American foundation for the blind, 1988.

Bibliography

Colenbrander A. Dimensions of visual performance. Trans Am Acad Ophthalmol Otolaryngol. 1977; 83: 22.

Evans NK. Access to vision rehabilitation services for older adults. Optom Vis Sci. 1993; 70 (suppl):164.

Gresset J, Baumgarten M. A survey of rehabilitation services by the visually impaired elderly population. In: Kooijman AC, Looijestijn PL, Welling JA, van de Wildt GJ, eds. Low vision. Research and new developments in rehabilitation. Amsterdam: IOS Press, 1994; 481-484.

Lovie-Kitchin JE. Low vision services in Australia. J Vis Impair Blind. 1990; 84: 298-304.

Lovie-kitchin JE, keeffe JE and Taylor HR. Referral to low vision services by optometrists. Clin Exp Optom. 1996; 79: 227-233.

Resnikoff S, Pascolini D, Etya'ale K, Pararajasegaram R, Pokharel G, Mariotti SP. Global data on visual impairment in the year 2002. Bull World Health Org. 2004; 82: 844-851.

Rosenbloom A A and Goodrich G. Visual rehabilitation: historic perspective future perspectives. In Johnston AW, Lawrence M, eds. Low vision ahead II: proceedings of the international conference on low vision. Melbourne: Association for the blind, 1990; 286-291.

World Health Organization (WHO). International classification of impairment, disabilities and handicaps: a manual of relationship to the consequences of diseases. Geneva. World Health Organization, 1980.

World Health Organization. Strategies for the prevention of blindness in national programmes. A primary health care approach. 2nd Ed. World Health Organization; Geneva1997.

Chapter 2
Impacts of Visual Impairment and Rehabilitation of the Visually Impaired

Reduced vision has a significant impact on daily activities of an individual. Many people may not be able to perform daily living activities due to poor visual acuity or visual field loss. Some may require high levels of lighting to be able to see well, while others, because of abnormal sensitivity to glare may require reduced level of illumination for task performance. Therefore, many people may not be able to function effectively under normal illumination level. Low vision due to visual impairment and associated environmental modification needs may affect many daily activities of an individual. Every activity that a person engages in, may be affected by low vision or blindness. One's vocation, hobby and even the activities of daily self-keeping are all affected by low vision. The following are some of the various categories of activities that may be affected by low vision.

For basic tasks such as reading and writing personal mail or knitting, a low vision patient will benefit from optical and non-devices. There are several optical and non-optical devices for these purposes, many of which are simple and relatively cheap. All that is needed is that the services are made available and patients be appropriately referred. These dictate the need for eye care practitioners to develop interest in low vision care and get more involved in the provision of rehabilitation services for individuals with low vision. Also, there is a dire need for low vision rehabilitation services to be established where they are not currently available, especially at government facilities. Prompt and appropriate referral to low vision services needs to be done by eye care practitioners and patients should be encouraged to utilize available services.

Effects on Vocational and Avocation Activities

A person with low vision will have difficulty performing vocational activities such as computer operation, driving, schooling et *cetera*. Also, she or he may have problems with recreational activities such as taking part in sports, reading novels, gardening and watching television. Attending social activities such as going to shopping, attending social gathering may be a problem due to poor acuity. Activities of daily living such as self-care, cooking and house-keeping may also present difficulties. A person with low vision will have difficulty performing vocational activities such as computer operation, driving, schooling et *cetera*. Also, she or he may have problems with recreational activities such as taking part in sports, reading novels, gardening and watching television. Attending social activities such as going to shopping, attending social gathering may be a problem due to poor acuity. Activities of daily living such as self-care, cooking and house-keeping may also present difficulties.

Blindness in terms of visual acuity loss or visual field loss or both often affects functional activities of a person more than low vision, therefore a blind person has greater difficulty in performing activities of daily living (ADL). In general terms, blindness affects all activities that are affected by low vision to a greater degree. All visually-guided tasks are adversely affected by blindness. The disability involved being directly related to the degree of blindness. If some form of vision still remains, the visual handicap may be less than when there is no light perception.

A few of these various impacts of visual impairment on affected individuals are thematically listed below, and briefly discussed below. Interestingly, these various impacts are interrelated, for example, inability to read and write is related to socio-economic impact, which on the other hand is related to psych-social and quality of life. Inability to move around impacts on socio-economic status and quality of life etc. Therefore, while it is possible to thematically list them, each domain cannot be considered in isolation.

Effects on Reading and Writing

Reading and writing are major activities of man in this modern age. Unfortunately, these are majorly affected by visual impairment, either as a consequence of visual acuity loss or visual field loss. Inability to read or write, even among literate persons, as a consequence of visual impairment would debar a person from many socio-economic activities. Children, especially those at school are particularly affected. Vision is a major sense for children, therefore visual impairment is a serious deterrent to their academic progress and life-long progress except appropriate rehabilitation is provided.

Effects on Locomotion and Environmental Navigation

Depending on the degree, vision or visual field loss affects locomotion hence environmental navigation. The blind persons seriously find moving around quite difficult irrespective of whether the impairment is due to visual acuity or visual field limitation. Climbing a step may present difficulty due to stereo-acuity loss associated with reduced vision. A person with visual impairment may find environmental navigation and independent travelling quite difficult or impossible unless assisted. Even, if the person has a car, has driving skill and may manage to drive. However, he may not be able to acquire a driver's license because of his or her visual impairment.

Impact on Social and Economic Status

A person who is visually-impaired may not be able to engage in social or economic activities independently, depending on the degree of the impairment. He or she may not be able to attend social gathering alone. For example, attending religious activities or cinema or sporting activities become difficult or impossible. This may lead to feeling of social isolation. Visual disability affects a person's QoL by limiting social interaction and independence.[1,2]. A visually impaired person may not be able to partake in vocations which dependent on vision. Many employers, may be unwilling to hire a visually impaired person. Even, if he gets employed, going to work alone may be impossible. Inability to work or to secure an employment would result in financial difficulties and dependence on family, friends, community or government for financial support. The visually impaired person, especially those with severe impairment may not be able to engage in many avocational activities such as playing golf, basketball, football et cetera, except appropriate rehabilitation is provided.

Effects Quality of Life

Generally, quality of life (QoL) describes a person's self-concept or perception of his or her well-being or life satisfaction in relation to his or her cultural or community expectations and the perception norms. This perception includes how satisfied he is, with aspects of his or her socio-economic and health status. The World Health Organization[3] defines quality of life as the individual's perception of his or her position in life in the context of the culture and value system in which they live and in relation to their goals, standards, expectations, and concerns Social and economic conditions, personal characteristics and values of norms of indigenous and local populations are all factors affecting the impact of disease and health problems on a person's daily activities and his or her QoL[4] Quality of life may be the most important outcome to assess, when considering the effectiveness of treatment in patients, especially those with chronic or incurable diseases, and has become a central outcome of treatment, prevention, and support[5].

Visual impairment has a substantial impact on quality of life; compared with other chronic conditions and seems to affect the health-related spoiling the quality of life more than diseases such as diabetic type two, coronary syndrome and hearing impairment, but less than stroke, multiple sclerosis, chronic fatigue syndrome, major depressive disorder and severe mental illness. There is a significant reduction in scores on the self-care and mobility domain of quality of life in individuals with tunnel vision. Individuals with visual field impairment experience a lower QoL and that the defects affecting the visual field decreases the persons QoL[6,7]

Quality of life is influenced by various factors such as social, economic, cultural and physical health[8] Income has a significant effects on QoL, with patients with low income having many psychological and other emotional problems. The impacts of employment, social presence, and financial independence as social determinants of health may improve QoL in individuals[9]

One of the important goals of rehabilitation programs is to assess and improve the QoL in individuals with disabilities. Rehabilitation program in all its ramifications is the only way to assist persons who are visually impaired. A comprehensive and holistic management approach is the current method of rehabilitation of the visually impaired.

A Holistic Rehabilitation of Visually Impaired Patients

Due to low vision, a patient would have difficulty performing many activities of daily living (ADL) and many other mundane activities therefore would require some form of rehabilitation programme to perform certain specific activities. Rehabilitation in relation to health care has been defined as a process of helping handicapped individuals move from positions of dependency toward positions of independence in a community of their choice[10] and this definition applies to low vision rehabilitation. Although, there is no possibility of reversing low vision, people with the condition can return to an active, productive rewarding and independent lifestyle following appropriate rehabilitation[11,12]. For the low vision patient, the lifestyle changes following rehabilitation may include achievement of visual goals, which may in turn lead to improvement in quality of life (QoL).

The rehabilitation of a person with low vision, requires a programme which involves holistic consideration of the person's social, economic, and psychological needs, rather than concentrating only on his or her visual needs. Low vision patients should be seen as a whole person having a range of physical and psychological needs[13]. This implies that apart from the visual needs, which can be met by Optometrists and Ophthalmologists, others concerns such as social, economic and psychological requirements need to be adequately addressed. Many are frustrated because they can no longer engage in simple activities such as reading and watching television, while others are become socially isolated because they can no longer travel independently or cannot attend social gathering.

Low vision can affect the quality of life of the person who has the condition. It has been reported that most patients would benefit significantly, from rehabilitation processes provided by the appropriate low vision service and would thus be able to improve their quality of life. Such programme relies on an interdisciplinary team of professionals and/or para-professionals to provide an effective service. The various professionals who could be part of the vision rehabilitation team include the optometrist, ophthalmologist, psychologist, psychiatrist, audiologist, social worker, occupational therapist, special educator, orientation and mobility instructor, reading specialist, visual therapist and physiotherapist. The role of each of these professionals is briefly discussed below.

Holistic Rehabilitation of Low Vision Patients

Due to low vision, the patient would have difficulty performing many activities of daily living (ADL) and would require rehabilitation programme. Although, there is no possibility of reversing the visual impairment, LVP can return to an active, productive, rewarding and independent lifestyle with low vision devices and re-habilitation training[11,12]. The re-habilitation of a person with low vision requires a programme which involves a holistic consideration of the person's social, economic and psychological needs rather than concentrating only on his or her visual needs.

Low vision can affect the quality of life of the person who has the condition. It has been reported that most patients would benefit from rehabilitation processes provided by the low vision service and would thus be able to improve their Quality of Life (QoL). Such programme relies on an interdisciplinary team of professionals or para-professionals to provide an effective service. The various professionals who could be part of the vision rehabilitation team include the optometrist, ophthalmologist, psychologist, psychiatrist, audiologist, social worker, occupational therapist, special educator, orientation and mobility instructor, reading specialist, visual therapist and physiotherapist. The role of each of these professionals is briefly discussed in this article.

Optometrist

Low vision care with respect to optometry, is a relatively new but rapidly growing field of eye care. A team approach, utilising the rehabilitation medicine approach, has been advocated by several authors and is still being developed. The optometrist is a part of the rehabilitation team concerned with helping the visually impaired patient function to his or her full potential. The optometrist is often the first professional that the low vision patient contacts in the rehabilitative team, and he or she is involved with the visual assessment, diagnosis of the cause, and the degree of visual disability.

Rehabilitation can change the quality of life of a visually impaired person; for instance, a person who otherwise may not be able to move around independently due to visual impairment may be able to do so after undergoing a visual examination, provision of a telescope and appropriate mobility training. Also, a person who is not able to read personal mail due to reduced vision, and had to depend on others for this task may on acquiring a magnifier (spectacle, hand or stand) of appropriate power and training, may be able to read such post independently. Further, a student who suddenly becomes visually impaired and therefore, is not able to continue his or her studies may be able to resume such studies after acquisition of relevant optical and/or electronic devices and training in their use. Furthermore, a person may lose his or her job as a result of low vision. With appropriate low vision devices, training and counselling, he or she may be able to secure another job. Optometrists therefore, have a great role to play in the rehabilitation of the low vision patient.

With regard to optometry, rehabilitation includes educating the patient about low vision, referral to community resources, teaching the client how to eccentrically view and read more effectively, the use of both optical and non-optical assistive devices, and in some cases sensory substitution for Activities of Daily Living (ADL). Many people with low vision are frustrated because they can no longer engage in simple activities such as reading their letters, while others feel socially isolated because they can no longer travel independently as they used to. Therefore, vision rehabilitation for patients with low vision can involve a range of services depending to a large extent, on the degree of vision loss. The services required may include programmes for independent living, the provision of assistive devices and training programmes, low vision therapy, orientation and mobility training, and creation of job opportunities for the visually impaired. Some of these activities can be provided by the optometrist. Once the patient has been referred to such a program, it is the duty of the multidisciplinary rehabilitation team to ensure the cooperation and active participation of the patient in the entire rehabilitation process.

Rehabilitation strategies for patients is considered to be functional-goal and attitude-oriented. The functional oriented strategy consists of providing the patients with assistive technology, teaching them the alternative strategies and recommending environmental modifications with the aim of helping them to achieve specific behavioural goals. The goal-oriented strategy, in turn, consists of assisting the patient to engage in specific behavioural activities (such as reading the newspaper) that the patient wants to perform but no longer can because of visual impairment. With regard to low vision, the functional and goal-oriented strategies are within the domains of the optometrist. The optometrist may also be able to provide some attitude-oriented strategies, but this is particularly within the domain of psychologists or psychiatrists.

Referral to other professionals, services or resources is one of the roles of the optometrist. Although optometry training includes caring for patients with low vision; not all optometrists engage in low vision care, therefore an optometrist may refer a low vision patient to another optometrist for further care. Depending on the ocular clinical findings, the optometrist who engages in low vision care, may refer the low vision patient to other professionals. In certain cases, referral and management by other professionals should take place before the optometric management is commenced because the assessment, treatment and rehabilitation outcome of one professional can influence the activities of the other. For instance, referral to the ophthalmologist for disease management should be done before optometric services are commenced, otherwise the use of low vision devices may not be successful. Also, low vision, like other disabilities is frequently associated with psychological, social and economic consequences; therefore, patients with low vision should be seen as a whole person having ranges of physical and psychological needs. Therefore, if there are indications of serious emotional reactions as a result of the vision loss, the patient may need to be referred for psychological management before optometric management.

The optometrist also often refers the low vision patients to other relevant services, particularly social services, orientation and mobility training, applications for financial assistance such as transport subsidies and disability support, if the eligibility criteria are met. A major role of the optometrist, is to prescribe appropriate low vision optical, electronic and/ or non-optical device/s which would enable the patient to achieve certain functional goal/s. Following the establishment that the patient is a low vision patient and absence of a need for a referral, the optometrist would examine the patient. The conventional pattern of basic vision assessment generally includes case history, visual acuity measurement, refraction (objective and subjective), ocular health evaluation, visual field, colour vision and contrast sensitivity assessments. This is followed by functional visual assessment in which the low vision devices that the person requires to perform desired tasks are determined. These could be optical or electronic devices for distance and or nearby. The powers of the devices and the distance, where each device will be, have to be determined. Quite often, a low vision patient would benefit from optical, electronic and non-optical devices; therefore more than one device may need to be prescribed.

Successful low vision rehabilitation involves more than prescribing low vision devices as it includes provision of instruction, training, and supportive services to enhance the patient's performance in the ADL. Whatever device that is prescribed for the patient, an appropriate training in their use has to be provided otherwise the patient will not benefit maximally from the device/s.

Further, a follow-up visit will have to be scheduled to ensure that the patient is complying with the mode of use, is using and benefiting from the devices. For many low vision patients, the provision of appropriate level of illumination can mean the difference between being able or unable to perform a visual task. The optometrist is also involved in the illumination control processes; hence they prescribe relevant filters and educate the patient on the appropriate level of illumination that will enhance their visual performance. Coloured filters are able to contribute substantially to rehabilitation of low-vision patients; they can lead to improved VA, contrast sensitivity function (CSF) for all frequencies; reduction in glare sensitivity, reduction of photophobia, eye-strain and eye discomfort.

The Optometrist is also involved in educating and advising the patient on the limitations of his vision. For instance he or she informs the patient if the vision does not meet the legal limits such as for driving. Even when a patient does not benefit from assistive devices, the optometrist still has a role to play. He or she may play an important but relatively minor role in the vision rehabilitation of patients with severe visual impairment, especially those with significant visual field loss. Referrals for counselling and social support are vital to assist such patients to manage their visual handicap. Practical assistance to help overcome their limitations in ADL is then more likely to be accepted.

Optometrists also plays a role in establishing a low vision patient's eligibility for rehabilitation, educational and recreational activities as the information from the eye examination has a role in establishing a patient's eligibility for both rehabilitation and education involvement. The optometrist therefore, can initiate the access to these facilities. People with low vision are usually apprehensive of going blind and this may result in emotional consequences. In this regard, the optometrist counsels the patient to help him or her to understand the present visual status, possible prognosis and what opportunities are available for low vision care. It is essential to let the patient know that there is no cure for his or her eye condition, but that low vision care can assist in using remaining vision to a certain degree and a comprehensive rehabilitation process would improve his or her quality of life.

Ophthalmologist

The ophthalmologist's role in eye care is fundamentally one of treatment, restoration, prevention and provision of information about the condition, its prognosis as well as referral for rehabilitation. The ophthalmologist is, therefore, involved in examining the patient and establishing the etiology of the low vision. He or she is also involved with the management of the pathological ocular conditions that may require medication or surgical intervention. He or she also decides the stability or otherwise, of the ocular disease. This is an important decision as optometric low vision care may not commence until there are indications that the eye or systemic disease resulting in low vision has stabilized The ophthalmologist is also involved with the recommendation of the patient for registration as a low vision patient and informing the patient about the nature of the disease and motivate them to start low vision care in order to improve their quality of life. In some countries, only the ophthalmologist can recommend a patient for registration as a low vision patient.

The ophthalmologist may also provide some education to the patient regarding the level and limitation of his vision and what services are available for rehabilitation. A few ophthalmologists may also be involved in prescribing optical, non-optical and electronic devices to low vision patients, but in most cases, patients are referred to an optometrist for provision of optical and non-optical devices. It has been reported that ophthalmologist can help improve the QoL for the patient with age-related macular degeneration by treating the patient and providing referral for psychiatric care for depression, especially if symptoms are persistent.

Psychologist and Psychiatrist

Low vision can be a traumatising experience, depending on several factors such as severity, suddenness, duration of the vision loss, the economic status, age and attitude of the person. For instance, a sudden vision loss can lead to emotional reaction such as shock and denial, which can eventually lead to depression. Low vision can leave a person anxious, depressed, confused or even fearful of his or her surroundings. The depression associated with low vision may be because the person can no longer partake in the activities that he or she used to do such as vocational, educational, recreational and social activities and Activities of Daily Living (ADL). The common incidence of depression among people with visual impairment has been associated with impaired visual and physical functions[13].

With loss of vision, a person finds that he or she has lost one of the main sensory organs and is no longer as independent as previously. In addition, loss of vision may sometimes result in loss of a job. Disability, handicap and frustration associated with visual impairment, therefore are often associated with psychological problems. The inability to perform ADL, decreased QoL and the reported increase in economic burden among this population may also be some of the reasons for the depression.

It has been reported that persons with low vision have a higher probability of concentration problems during reading and entertainment, losing interest and enjoyment in their activities, feeling fatigued, irritable, sad, and tearful; having less hope for the future and wishing for death. There is association between visual impairment and perceived low level of happiness in life, difficult periods or crisis and symptoms of distress such as depression, sleeping difficulties and tiredness, intrusive thoughts especially about vision, isolation and loneliness, worries and tension, distress about economic conditions, poor health attribution and depressive feelings. It has been proposed that, since attitudes are culturally determined, the loss of vision may threaten a person's integrity.

Beaty[14] hypothesized that visual impairment may lead to feelings of inadequacy and inferiority which may result in self-concept deficit. In a similar study, Obiakor and Stile[15], however, did not find such self-concept deficit among adolescents with visual impairments. It is, therefore, possible that self-concept deficit is not a general finding among individuals with visual impairment. The difference may be related to the environment in which an individual finds himself. For instance, a low vision patient who works among other low vision patients is less likely to exhibit a work-related negative self-concept, but another patient who works among normally sighted individuals may exhibit such a concept, especially if the co-workers are critical of him or her. A psychologist or psychiatrist can therefore be of help in cases where there is an associated psychological manifestation of poor self-concept.

Low vision and loss of ability to perform ADL result in decline of quality of life (QoL). The deterioration in QoL has been associated with increase in the degree of visual impairment (VI) and presumably may also be a consequence of the economic burden that has been associated with visual impairment. The presence or absence of psychological problems may be influenced by personality factors, severity and type of onset (sudden or gradual) of the condition. The nature of the condition such as suddenness, gradual and steadily deteriorating, or fluctuating may elicit emotional reactions. For the visually impaired persons not to suffer psychological disorders, the person should positively adapt to the new situation using positive strategies such as acceptance, trust, positive avoidance, minimization and control.

When low vision patients show exacerbating emotional or psychological reactions, their rehabilitation will not be complete without the assistance of a clinical psychologist, psychotherapist or a psychiatrist who will deal with such problems, which have to be dealt with along with the visual problems. The visually impaired persons need psychological support at two levels in the rehabilitation process: the emotional level and the level of coping with daily activities. These two levels of support are provided by the Psychologist or Psychiatrist whose modes of operation include counselling or psychotherapy. Some psychologists are involved in skills training for the low vision patients. Visually, impaired children and adolescents and their families are at a high risk for maladjustment and distress, and in such cases, the psychologists can help in parent-child problems solving interactions in the families.

Attitude oriented strategy of rehabilitation is mainly in the hands of the psychologist and psychiatrist and may involve helping the patient to adjust psychologically to the limitations imposed by the impairments and this may involve counselling the patient to surrender unrealistic goals, learn to accept the current situation and face the challenges imposed by the visual impairment[12]. They need to be assisted in gaining a new perspective, to re-evaluate their goals, and to accept the challenges imposed by the visual impairment. Also, people with low vision need counselling in order to have hope for the future in spite of the current changes in their visual status. They need to be informed that there is a possibility of improvement in their quality of life, in spite of their reduced vision. In view of the various psychological associated with low vision, the psychologist and psychiatrists are important components of low vision rehabilitation.

Audiologist

In Dual Sensory Impairment (DSI), visual disability is associated with hearing loss; hence the audiologist may be involved in low vision rehabilitation. DSI may present at any age as a result of genetic defect, accident, injury, disease or environmental insults. This condition has wide range implications for physical and psychological functioning and quality of life. In Usher's syndrome, a genetic condition, retinitis pigmentosa is accompanied by hearing loss. With hearing loss, subjective refraction may be difficult. Hearing may be aided by modern electronic aids or hearing assisted telephones.

The problems encountered by individuals with DSI are considerably greater than the effects of vision impairment or hearing impairment alone, because when these two sensory impairments are combined, the individual is seriously deprived of compensatory strategies that make use of the non-impaired sense. Cochlear implant can play a significant rehabilitative role in patients with severe hearing loss and visual impairment. About two-thirds of patients with age-related macular degeneration (AMD) have visuomotor and balance deficits resulting in clumsiness and increased risk of falls. Visual, vestibular and somatosensory functions in balance control can be rehabilitated by training. This may result in a significant improvement for the vestibular input and fixation stability including postural sway, pointing accuracy, reading performance.

Social Worker

Low vision can lead to loss of job or inability to secure employment, therefore has social and economic implications. The implication for the patient in terms of job, pension *et cetera* must be considered. Also, the effects of visual performance on dependency relationships and family role have to be kept in mind. While the immediate situation must be dealt with, the patient's long term adjustment to his or her disability is often more important. Therefore, a social worker may be needed for counselling and to search for an appropriate alternative employment. Also, the social worker can play an important role in both the evaluation and treatment of the patient with low vision. Social workers can participate in the psychosocial assessment, and help assess the client's coping and adaptation to the vision loss. Vision impairment has been associated with depression. An important role for the social worker in rehabilitation is to provide referral for counselling services.

The social worker is also knowledgeable about community and government resources as well as potential financial assistance. Providing guidance and education about these issues may lead to more effective adaptation and coping with the vision impairment. People with low vision need hope and need to know that their quality of life can improve, even though their vision is not as good as it used to be. They need to be informed of how adaptive devices and low vision services can help them use remaining vision more effectively. In addition, their families need to be informed about how they can support their loved ones with low vision. The social worker can effectively play this role.

The social workers can also guide the patient through the rehabilitation process by way of encouraging the patient, particularly when he or she needs to try tasks or activities which are new or threatening or for which the person has low confidence. Also, assisting job seekers with disabilities to find jobs is an important part of rehabilitation. The social worker can also assist in the assessment of whether or not the devices prescribed for the patient is being used. Counselling may be required before some patients will accept referral or advice regarding practical solutions to overcome their limitations in ADL. Assistance with ADL and counselling can also be provided too by the social worker. Therefore, a multi-disciplinary approach to the management of low vision and blindness should include the social worker.

Occupational Therapist

The occupational therapist is involved in the assessment, recommendation and provision of equipment. He or she is also concerned with providing and instructing people in the use of the equipment in solving his or her vocational and avocational and functional problems[16]. Occupational therapy as a profession entered the field of low vision rehabilitation (LVR) only recently, being preceded by orientation and mobility (O&M) specialists, low vision therapists, and teachers of the visually impaired. OTs started working in LVR in the United States sometime after 1990 and a similar situation subsequently developed in Canada with a handful of OT practitioners applying LVR. Occupational therapy offers a programme that specializes in the assisting people with low vision. Restoring and maintaining the ability of the low vision patient to function independently through the use of specific interventions is an intricate process that calls for the collaboration of various health care professionals and occupational therapists (OTs) are essential members of the multidisciplinary rehabilitation team providing such interventions. The role of the occupational therapist includes determination of the cognitive, psychosocial, and physical needs of the client. The evaluation process allows the occupational therapist to evaluate visual and non-visual client factors, history, roles, physical environment, and occupational performance. Based on the evaluation, the therapist will design a vision rehabilitation program to teach the client how to function more effectively in ADLs in spite of the vision loss.

In low vision rehabilitation, OTs can enhance performance of specific activity of daily living (ADL) by training skills that are dependent on residual vision such as reading and writing. They also conduct environmental assessments in the home and in the workplace or school to improve and promote a safe environment for patients with low vision. The OTs may also assist in developing rehabilitation programs for orientation and mobility, driving, and vision rehabilitation therapy. When there is a difficulty in coping with daily living activities, the OT has to train the patient on alternate methods, in the use of assistive devices, modify environment and educate the patient and the family on coping strategies. This approach may lead to increased level of independence, improved safety, increased adequacy of performance and decreased difficulty and increased satisfaction.

Occupational therapists may be involved in the assessment, recommendation and provision of assistive devices and instructing people in the use of the devices in solving the patient's specific vocational, avocational and functional problems. During the occupational therapy evaluation, two parameters of activity, namely safety and independence are emphasized. This will help the patient perform ADL independently and safely. Management of lighting, contrast, and glare are also critical roles of the therapist. The occupational therapist may need to refer the client to the low vision optometrist if he/she finds that the client may benefit from low vision devices or the prescribed optical, non-optical or electronic devices are not as effective as desired. In addition, the occupational therapist may assist where a patient requires training in the use and adjustment to the optical devices and non-optical devices. For a new employment, there is usually a need for training in the use of the various equipment in the workplace to ensure independence and safety, and this training may be done by the OT.

Special Educators

The eye is an important organ for learning as a large proportion of what a child learns is via the eye and the visual system. Children who are visually impaired are potentially at a great disadvantage academically unless a special educational system is provided. Many children with visual impairment receive education at specialized schools for the blind where, besides the core curriculum, they were taught adaptive skills. Special educational system requires special teachers and special learning materials as well as necessary environmental modifications.

The partially sighted children need teachers who understand their visual limitations and demands and who have the special knowledge required for their social and educational circumstances and needs. Children who are blind and/or visually impaired must be allowed to learn compensatory skills to achieve therapeutic goals. Development of these skills can be accomplished most effectively when these children receive services from qualified specialists in a team setting. Special educators are specifically trained to meet the social, educational and developmental needs of children with various types of disabilities. These teachers occupy an important position in the rehabilitation process of the children as they are usually the link between the child and other rehabilitation professionals.

Orientation and Mobility (O&M) Instructor

Orientation and mobility (O&M) is a set of skills that allow persons with visual impairments to move safely efficiently and gracefully, know their location and remain orientated in their environment during travel. These skills are taught by O&M specialists[17]. The orientation and mobility instructor is an important professional in the rehabilitation of the visually disabled. Many low vision patients do not need orientation and mobility, there are, however, a few who may need such training. The OM instructor teaches the low vision and blind persons how to move around freely in their environment, by introducing them to certain landmarks in the environment which they then use for navigation.

An important aspect of orientation and mobility training may be in cases of those with severe peripheral field loss, therefore need training in environmental navigation. The O&M instructor may also train the person in performing certain ADLs in the environment. This rehabilitation process is necessary each time a visually disabled patient locates into a new environment such as new school, new work place or new accommodation and helps to minimize the frustration associated with the visual loss with regard to environmental navigation.

Physiotherapist

There are a variety of ways in which vision modulates locomotion in a feedback manner. Vision loss affects primarily stability aspect of gait, reducing the patient's ability to modify gait in response to obstacles in the environment. Also, visual inputs are an important source of information for postural control. Balance has been shown to be more impaired with greater visual impairment which could result in fall and injury and visual impairment has been reported to increase the risk of fall. These highlight the importance of physiotherapeutic role in the rehabilitation of the visually impaired. Physiotherapy can contribute to both the assessment and intervention programmes of the visually impaired.

Motor development and associated postural reactions will be trained, abnormal postures prevented or decreased, and body image and use of residual vision developed. Selection and supervision of devices and play equipment, as well as decreasing of physical handicap are also included in the physiotherapist's role in helping the child and his family. It has been recognized that motor training programmes such as balance, coordination, strength, visuomotor control, and finger dexterity improved skills of children with low vision.

Children with low vision have some useable vision and learning to use the available vision depends on proper rehabilitation including physiotherapy management. Children and elderly with visual impairment can therefore benefit from motor training provided by the physiotherapist. Since visual impairment may increase risk of falling, the physiotherapist will also be helpful in caring for the visually impaired persons who sustain injury as a result of falling due to visual impairment.

Reading Specialist

Low vision presents numerous challenges to the affected person, for many, it is difficulty with reading. Reading is a major desire of many low vision patients[18]. Many want to read newspapers while others wish to read religious books such as the bible. Unfortunately, even with necessary devices, reading with low vision requires more efforts than needed by the normally sighted persons. Also, reading with low vision requires certain compromises such as reading at a very short distance such as 25 cm or even closer. Low vision affects many aspects of reading, for instance, it is usually associated with a decreased reading speed, even when the optimum reading size is used. The person with low vision may require a higher or lower than normal level of illumination for reading, depending on the etiology of his or visual condition. He or she may need to turn the book upside down and read from right to left due to visual field defect and may require the use of electronic adaptive devices such as the closed circuit television (CCTV). These require special training and a reading specialist may be quite helpful.

A considerable variation has been observed in the results of studies in reading performance of people with visual impairment and this has been attributed to several factors. These factors include whether eye movements are required to scan along a line of print, whether the text is scanned across a CCTV screen, size of the print relative to acuity, whether unrelated words or continuous text is used, and pathology of the group studied and experience of the subject[19]. A reading specialist is required where there are indications of difficulty in achieving the desired reading ability with prescribed devices. The type of optical devices employed for reading also affects the process of reading. Compared to ordinary reading (without magnification), one might expect magnification of the text and the limited reading field to give rise to difficulties when reading with the aid of a magnifier. In view of the above, a reading specialist needs to be involved in the rehabilitation of the low vision patient.

Low Vision Therapist

Low vision therapy is one of the most recent development in the area of low vision care and also the most difficult to describe. The Certified Low Vision Therapist (CLVT) works as part of an interdisciplinary team with an ophthalmologist or optometrist who provides low vision care. The CLVT performs functional low vision evaluation relating to activities of daily living, educational and vocational pursuits, leisure, social activities, access and participation in community programmes, coping ability and impact of the vision disability on other relevant people[16]. He or she uses functional vision evaluation instruments to assess visual functions such as visual acuity, visual fields, contrast sensitivity function, colour vision, stereopsis, visual perceptual and visual motor functioning as well as literacy skills in reading and writing, as they relate to visual impairment and disability.

The low vision therapist may train the visually impaired person in the use of specific visual motor skills, such as the identification and use of preferred retinal locus for fixation, accurate saccades, and smooth pursuits as well as the use of appropriate environmental modifications such as positioning, organization, illumination control and marking. The CLVT also educates the family of the visually impaired and other relevant persons on the functional implications of vision and refers patients to other professionals in the rehabilitation team.

Success of Rehabilitation Services

A successful rehabilitation programme may reduce the rehabilitation demand by reducing the level of difficulty associated with the goal or task and/or by reducing the value assigned to the goal or task. Effective rehabilitation processes can make a lot of difference in the quality of life (QoL) of the low vision patient. Following an evaluation of the effectiveness of a multidisciplinary low vision rehabilitation, in which first time low vision referrals were assessed before and after 3-6 months rehabilitation, significant improvements were found in the impact of impairment score, reading, accessing information and emotional well-being. This confirms that effective low vision rehabilitation can greatly improve the quality of life (QoL) of the low vision patient. It is incumbent on those providing rehabilitation of the disabled persons to measure the effectiveness of such care.

Quality of life is an important outcome used in the evaluation of rehabilitation provided to individuals[20]. Improvement in QoL is often given as a major goal for therapy. The factors that have been used for defining QoL in relation to rehabilitation include social utility or the opportunity to fulfil valued social roles including work, emotional states such as happiness, satisfaction with one's own life conditions, achievement of personal goals and normal life measure by comparing current status to either pre-health or pre-illness condition. In low vision rehabilitation, clinical outcomes such as visual acuity in relation to visual performance achieved with the low vision devices or the usage of the devices have been used in the evaluation of low vision rehabilitation.

The factors that have been used for defining quality of life in relation to rehabilitation in general include the following[21].

i. Social utility or the opportunity to fulfil valued social roles including work

ii. Emotional states such as happiness
iii. Satisfaction with one's own life conditions
iv. Achievement of personal goals
v. Normal life measured by comparing current status to either pre-health or pre-illness condition.

Task performance such as the ability to read television titles or newspaper texts and questionnaires on low vision devices and satisfaction rates have also been used to assess quality of life. There is currently a strong case for using a wide range of outcome measures which should include task performance (ability to perform certain ADL) and a measure of psychological adjustment to visual loss in addition to vision specific measures. Effective rehabilitation of the low vision patient demands that a multidisciplinary approach be used. This implies that all relevant professionals should be involved in the rehabilitation of the patient. When necessary, every professional involved in the rehabilitation should involve other relevant ones so that the desired level of rehabilitation can be achieved. With this approach, the frustration that is inherent in low vision can be avoided and a better quality of life can be enjoyed by the patient.

References

1. Klein BE, Klein R, Lee KE, Cruickshanks KJ. Performance-based and self-assessment measures of visual function as related to history of falls, hip fracture, and measure of gait time. The Beaver Dam Eye Study. Ophthalmol. 1998; 105: (1); 160-164.
2. West SK, Munoz B, Rubin GS, Schein OD, Bandeen-Roche K, Zeger S, et al. Function and visual impairment in a population-based study of older adults. The SEE project Salisbury Eye Evaluation. Invest Ophthalmol Vis Sci. 1997; 38: (1); 72-82.
3. World Health Organization Quality of life Group (1993). Measuring quality of life: the development of the WHOQOL instrument, Geneva, Switzerland: world Health Organization; 1993. Available from: http://www.who.int/mental_health /media /68.pdf. Accessed 14 Feb, 2014.
4. Warrian KJ, Speath GL, Lankaranian D, Lopes JF, Steinmann WC. The effect of personality on measures of quality of life related to vision in glaucoma patients. Br J Ophthalmol. 2009; 93: (3); 310-315.
5. Lindholt JS, Ventegodt S, Hanneberg EW. Development of quality of life for clinical databases. A short global and generic questionnaire based on an integrated theory of the quality of life. Eur. J Surg. 2002; 168: 107-13.

McKeen-Cowdin R, Varma R, Wu, J, Hays RD, Azen SP. Loss Angeles Latino Eye Study Group. Severity of visual field and Health-related quality of life. Am J Ophthalmol. 2007; 143: (6); 1013-1023.

Patino CM, Varma R, Azen SP, Conti DV, Nichol MB, McKeen_Cowdin R et al. The impact of change in visual filed loss and health-related quality of Life. The Los Angeles Latino Eye Study. Ophthalmology. 2011; 118 (7): 1310-1317other chronic diseases. Ophthal Epidemiol. 2007; 14: (3) ;119-126.

Rubin SE, Chan F, Thomas DL. Assessing changes in life skills and quality of life resulting from rehabilitation services. J Rehab.2003; 69 (3): 4.Wexler DJ, Grant RW, Wittenberg E, Bosch JL, Cagliero E, Delahanty L et al. Correlates of health-related quality of life in type 2 diabetes. Diabetologica. 2006; 49: (7); 1489-11489-1497.

9. Khorrami-Nejadi M Sarabandi A, Akbarri Mohammed-Reza, Askarizadeh, F. The impact of visual impairment on Quality of life.

10. Emener WG, Hollingsworth DK. (Eds). Critical issues in rehabilitational counselling. Springfield. IL; Charles C Thomas. 1984.

Massof RW. A systems model for low vision rehabilitation. I. Basic Concepts. Optom. Vis Sci. 1995; 72: 725-736.

Kupfer C. The low vision education programme: Improving quality of life. Optom. Vis Sci. 1999; 76: 729-730.

Bairstow M. Low Vision: Social and rehabilitation needs. Optician. 1998; 216: 18-21.

Beaty LA. Adolescent self-concept as a function of vision loss. Adolescent 1992; 27:707-714.

Obiakor FE, Stile SW. Enhancing self-concept in students with visual handicaps, J Vis Impair Blind 1989; 83:255-257.

Moore M. Multi-disciplinary low vision care. Optician. 1994; 208: 24-27.

Balashova Y. First orientation and mobility teacher preparation programme in Russia. Intern Congr Series. 2005; 1282: 789-792.

Bower AR Reid VM. Eye movements and reading with simulated visual impairment. Ophthal Physiol Opt. 1997; 17: 392-402.

Leat JL and Woodhouse JM.22 Reading performance with low vision aids: relationship with contrast sensitivity. Ophthal Physiol. Opt. 1993; 13: 9-16.

Day H. Quality of life: Counterpoint. Can. J. Rehab. 1993; 6: 135-142.

Ferran H. Conceptualization of quality of life in cardiovascular research. Progress in cardiovascular nursing,

Bibliography

Aki E, Atasavun S, Turan A and Kayihan H. Training motor skills for children with low vision. Percept Mot Skills. 2007; 104: 1328-1336.

Andresen EM, Meyers AR. Health-related quality of life outcomes measures. Arch Phys Med Rehabil. 2000; 81 Suppl 2: S30-S45.

Aspinall PA, Johnson ZK, Azuara-blanco A, Montarzino A, Brice R, Vickers A. Evaluation of quality of life and priorities of patients with glaucoma. Invest Ophthalmol. 2008; 49: 1907-1915.

Bower AR Reid VM. Eye movements and reading with simulated visual impairment. Ophthal Physiol Opt. 1997; 17: 392-402.

Brennan M, Bally SJ. Psychosocial adaptations to dual sensory loss in middle and late adulthood. Trend Amplif, 2007; 11: 281-300.

Burlingham D. Some problems of ego development in blind children. Psychoanalyt study of child. 1965; 20: 194-208.

Cochrane G, Lamoureux E, Keeffe J. Defining the content for a new quality of life questionnaire for students with low vision (the impact of vision impairment on children. Ophthal Epidemiol. 2008 15: 114-120.

Esteban JJ, Martínez, MS, Navalon PG, Serrano OP, Patiño JR, Purón ME, Martínez-Vizceaíno V. Visual impairment and quality of life: gender differences in the elderly in Cuenca, Spain. Qual Life Res 2008; 17: 37-45.

Fabian ES and Waugh C. A job development efficacy scale for rehabilitation professionals. J Rehab. 2001; 67: 42-47.

Grover LL. Strategy for developing an evidence-based transdisciplinary vision rehabilitation team approach to treating vision impairment. Optom. 2008; 79: 178-188Holm M, Rogers J and James A. Interventions for daily living. In Crepeau EB,

Corn ES, and Boyt SB. Willard and Spackman's occupational therapy. Philadelphia: Lippincott, Willaims and Wilkins, 2003 pp 494-661.

Kern T. Barbier AC, Feist N. Integrated rehabilitation for the visually impaired, physically challenged children. Intern Congr Series. 2005; 1282: 179-183.

Heyman KJ, Kerse NM, La Grow SJ, Wouldes T, Robertson MC, Campbell AJ. Depression in older people: Visual impairment rating of health. Optom Vis Sci. 2007; 84: 1024-30.

Karlsson JS. Self-report of psychological distress in connection with various degrees of visual impairment. J Visual imp and blindness. 1998; 92: 483-491.

Lamoureux EL, Pallant JF, Pesudovs K, Rees G, Hassell JB and Keefe JE. The effectiveness of low vision rehabilitation on participation in daily living and quality of life. Invest Ophthalmol Vis Sci. 2007; 48; 1476-1482.

Leat JL, Woodhouse JM. Reading performance with low vision aids: relationship with contrast sensitivity. Ophthal Physiol Opt. 1993; 13 9-16.

Lee HKM, Skudds RJ. Comparison of balance in older people with and without visual impairment. Age and aging. 2003; 32: 643-649.

Legge GE, Pelli DG, Rubin GS, Schleske MM. Psychophysics of reading: Low Vision. Vision Res. 1985; 25: 239-252.

Markowitz M. occupational therapy intervention in low vision rehabilitation. Can J Ophthalmol. 2006; 41: 340-347.

Mojon-Azzi SM, Souza-Posa A, Mojon DS. Impact of low vision on well-being in 10 European Countries. Ophthalmologica. 2008; 222, 205: 212.

Nguyen NX, Weisemenan M, Trauzettel-klosinski S. Spectrum of ophthalmologic and social rehabilitation at the Tübinger low vision clinic: A retrospective analysis of 1999-2005. Ophthalmol. 2008; 105: 563-569

Oduntan, AO. Rehabilitation of visually impaired students in an institution of tertiary education. S. Afr Optm. 2003 63 3-9.

Okamoto F, Okamoto Y, Hiraoka T, Oshika T. Vision related quality of life and visual function after retinal detachment surgery. Am J Ophthalmol. 2008; 146: 85-90.

Otterstedde C R, Spandau U, Blankenagel A, Kimberling W J, Reisser C. A new clinical classification for Usher's syndrome based on a new subtype of Ushers's syndrome type I. Laryngoscope. 2001; 111: 84-6.

Radvav X, Duhoux S, Koenig-Supiot F, Vital-Durand F. Balance training and visual rehabilitation of age-related macular degeneration patients. J Vestib Res. 2007; 17: 183-193.

Rovner BW, Casten RJ, Tasman WS. Effect of depression on vision function in age-related macular degeneration. Arch Ophthalmol. 2002; 120:1041-1044.

Saunders GH, Echt KV. An overview of dual sensory impairment in older adults: perspectives for rehabilitation. Trends Amplif. 2007: 11: 243-258.

Scheiman M. Low vision rehabilitation. A practical guide for Occupational therapist. New Jersey, Professional Books, 2007.

Stelmark J. Emergence of a rehabilitation medicine model for low vision service delivery, policy and funding. Optom. 2005; 76: 318-326.

Sykanda AM, levitt S. The physiotherapist in the developmental management of the visually impaired child: Care, Health and Development. 2006 8: 261-270.

Tasman W, Rovner B. Age-related macular degeneration: treating the whole patient. Can J Ophthalmol. 2005; 40: 389-391.

Chapter 3
Clinical Assessment of Adult Low Vision Patients

A major consequence of low vision is the inability to perform visually guided activities such as reading, driving, watching television, shopping *et cetera*. Examination of a low vision patient is a functional assessment to determine if the visual acuity or visual field that he or she has can be enhanced to enable him or her to perform the specific task or tasks that he or she wishes to perform. The examination procedures are generally similar to that of the normally sighted patient, but there are certain specific differences due to the low level of vision and the psychological issues that may be involved low vision cases. The procedures commonly used in the basic assessment of low vision patients include general observation of the patient, visual acuity measurement, case history, external examination, disease diagnosis, refraction as well as binocular, contrast sensitivity, visual field, and colour vision assessments. All these procedures may not be applicable to every patient. The tests chosen depend on the visual condition of the patient, his or her the specific visual need and the assessment method of the practitioner.

The Low Vision Clinic Room

Apart from the usual optometric equipment used for examining the normally sighted patients, a low vision clinic requires additional equipment, for example low vision distance acuity chart which is able to measure acuity as low as 6/360 acuity. A commonly used chart is the Feinbloom distance acuity chart. Standard Bailey and Lovie distance acuity chart or similar charts are useful. The near charts should include low vision letter, words, and paragraph reading acuity charts. The Bailey word-reading charts are particularly useful in the evaluation of reading ability of low vision patients. There should be a wide range of optical and non-optical low vision devices as well. The optical devices should include spectacle magnifiers, hand-held, and stand magnifiers. Also, various types of telescopes (monocular, binocular, hand held, and face worn should be available. Where possible, close circuit television (CCTV) and other electronic devices should be available. As electronic devices are expensive, they may not be part of mandatory devices for starting a low vision practice. They can be purchased later, as they are important components of a standard low vision practice.

The Low Vision Care Patient

The type of low vision patient being dealt with depends on several factors such as the referral source, the age, the level of motivation, the purpose for which low vision aid is being sought. Following a routine refraction or basic vision assessment, if the practitioner finds that the patient has low vision, he or she may have to schedule the patient for low vision examination and management if necessary. A new low vision patient may be difficult to deal with, if he or she has the impression that his or her vision can be ameliorated by routine refraction and the provision of eyeglasses. He or she may therefore, not be mentally prepared for low vision devices. There may be a need to educate him or her about his or her vision status and prepare his or her mind for low vision care.

The level of motivation of the patient needs to be evaluated first before low vision care is commenced. If there is an indication that the patient had accepted the diagnosis of his or her vision status and agreed to try low vision low vision devices, a low vision examination should be commenced or scheduled for him or her. An indication of non-acceptance of the low vision status suggests that low vision care should be delayed till such time when the patient is motivated enough for such service. A patient who has previous knowledge of his low vision status and has accepted the situation favourably may be easier to deal with. Those who have tried low vision devices or those who have previously rejected low vision devices but have decided to have them now, are very good candidates for low vision care. Those who have specific purposes for which they are seeking low vision devices are also very good low vision care candidates compared to those who just want to improve their vision.

Pre-examination Instructions

A patient who is scheduled for low vision examination should be advised to bring all previous and current spectacles and optical devices that he or she may currently be using, or had used in the past. These will help the practitioner to know what devices that the patient currently uses, or is conversant with, or had knowledge of using. Any document relating to previous medical or eye examination, if available, should be brought on the examination day. These will provide some information about the systemic and ocular health of the patient. The patient may at this stage be asked to provide contact details of his or her medical or eye care practitioner. A casual observation of the patient should be made and those who may not be able to provide the necessary information that may be needed by the low vision practitioner or who may not be able to respond adequately to questions from the practitioner should be advised to come with a family member or a friend to assist in answering relevant questions. Low vision assessment can be time consuming, therefore an estimated duration of the examination should be communicated to the patient at this stage. The envisaged cost of the visual examination and optical devices may also be discussed at this stage for the patient to know how to prepare for the assessment.

The Examination

Before the commencement of the low vision examination, the practitioner should have a good knowledge of the patient's ocular and medical history as well as other relevant information about the patient. The visual needs and previous and current optical or non-optical devices should be known. Therefore, before meeting the patient the practitioner must review whatever document or information that is available about him or her. These will help in communicating more effectively with the patient. The more the information that is available, the greater the chances of communicating with the patient effectively, efficiently, and responsibly.

The low vision examination may be broken into primary and secondary assessments. The first assessment will be to obtain baseline refractive and ocular health information about the patient. This will allow the examiner to gain an insight into the low vision devices that the patient might need or referral to an ophthalmologist for medical management prior to further low vision assessment. The second and subsequent visits may involve the evaluation of the patient for low vision optical, non-optical devices and environmental modification needs. The tests to be conducted on the first and subsequent visits will depend on the examiners mode of practice, ocular status of the patient as well as the visual and functional needs of the patient. It is important to establish who made the appointment for the patient. If the patient made the appointment, this may be indicative of his or her level of motivation to improve his or her vision. If the appointment was made by a family member or a friend, it is possible that this fellow who booked the appointment is the one seeking improvement in vision for the patient. In that case, it may be difficult to judge the motivation of the patient regarding improvement of his or her vision.

General Observation

At the first visit of a low vision patient, there is a need to observe the patient as he or she enters the consulting room. This provides the opportunity to evaluate the patient in terms of the degree of visual disability, accompanying physical and mental disability and possibly, the cause of visual impairment and disability. Some of the observations to be made and documented include the following:

Mobility

Whether the patient moves around, independently or assisted; fast or slow *et cetera*

Visual Status and Capability

Whether the patient easily recognizes his or her pathway, wears dark shade or not *et cetera*.

Posture

Body and head posture should be observed and noted as they assist in guiding the management of the patient.

Fixation

Any sign of eccentric fixation suggestive of strabismus or other forms of binocular dysfunction or visual field loss should be noted as these may be a pointer to the disorder of the case.

Physical disability

Any sign of physical disability, such as partial paralysis should be noted. These may also guide management of the patient.

Psychological State

Insight may be gained into the psychological state of the low vision patient with the observation of the facial expression of the patient. Attitude and motivation of the patient may be estimated. Any sign of aggression or unhappiness should be noted. These may guide the need for referral for counselling

These general observations of the patient should continue and documented throughout the visual examination of the patient as well as during the trial of the devices.

Case History

The case history is an important aspect of low vision evaluation and differs from that of a normally sighted patient because issues relating to the social, economic and psychological aspects of the patient's daily living are often a part of the history. The case history is an opportunity for the patient to relate with the eye care professional. The examiner must therefore, convey a caring attitude. The practitioner needs to show that he or she understands the concerns and needs of the patient. The case history therefore, gives the patient and the optometrist the opportunity to communicate in a cordial, frank, and confidential manner. Also, the case history helps the examiner to formulate a management focus. The various visual problems of the patient as well as the specific assistance required from the low vision practitioner should be clearly established during the case history.

While the practitioner dictates the direction and tempo of the case history, the patient must be given the opportunity to adequately express his or her opinion, feelings and concerns as much as possible. The examiner should try to adjust to the tempo of the patient; and with regard to an elderly patient the case history should proceed as slowly as possible. This will help to avoid frustrating the patient. As with the normally sighted patients, the case history is an ongoing procedure therefore, during the course of the examination, any relevant information must be obtained from the patient and added to the existing ones.

The tenure of case history also enables the optometrist to further observe the patient and come to certain tentative conclusions about his or her motivation as well as mental and emotional status. The examiner must ensure that the patient understands him or her properly, and time must be taken to observe him carefully. The type of personality characteristics as well as the pattern of behaviour exhibited by the patient must be carefully observed and documented as these will help to judge how the subsequent examination would proceed. Observations made previously should, where necessary, be confirmed with the patient during the case history. For instance, if the posture of the patient suggested photophobia, the patient will be able to confirm this. If facial scars were observed, the patient should be made to shed light on when and how the scar occurred.

The attitude of the patient to the visual loss should be evaluated during the case history. Is the patient communicative easily, effectively or not? Is there any indication that he or she is trying to select information suggestive of trying to conceal certain information? Generally, patients tend to be ambivalent and feel reluctant to divulge personal information, some of which may be useful for low vision practitioner. The patient should be persuaded to talk about the unusual aspects of his or her vision such as experiencing flashing lights, moving objects in the visual field or coloured patches, and where relevant, should be re-assured that these are common occurrences in individuals with low vision, especially elderly patients with the condition.

The observations of the practitioner here may give an indication of the problems that may be encountered in the subsequent procedures. The case history not only gives the practitioner the opportunity to evaluate the patient, but also provides the patient the opportunity to evaluate the practitioner in terms of how caring and dedicated he or she is. Generally patients tend to be appreciative of the practitioner's readiness and ability to help them to adjust to their present visual circumstances. The practitioner must, therefore, try to convince the patient that he or she understands the problems of the patient and is ready to offer the desired assistance to the best of his or her ability. The practitioner must be straightforward in his or her questions. Ambiguous statements must be avoided and the patient must be listened to attentively.

The patient must be given enough time to narrate his or her complaints or respond adequately to the question that he or she had been asked. He or she must be allowed to present his or her problem as fully as he or she wishes. It must be remembered that low vision patients differ, even when they present with similar visual problems. While some try to conceal their physical, systemic and visual problems in order to preserve some sense of integrity and dignity, others may exaggerate them in order to convince the eye care practitioner that they are in dire need of assistance. The examiner must thus endeavour to minimize his or her prejudices and knowledge about the patient's problem. He or she must not allow his or her knowledge of the patient's case overshadow or curtail the information being presented by the patient. The practitioner must, therefore, make judgement and decision on the case, not only on his or her knowledge, but also on the information presented by the patient.

The major areas of interest that the practitioner should try to establish is the main concern of the patient in terms of his or her visual needs or wants. Therefore, the main assistance he or she expects from the practitioner must be clearly established. Also, the cause and duration of the visual disorder must be determined. Those with long duration of low vision (two years or more) are likely to accept low vision devices more readily, than those who lost their normal vision a short while before. Those with recent vision loss may not be interested in trying low vision devices as they may still be thinking of the possibility of restoration of their vision by medical or spiritual means. Contrarily, those who lost their vision for a long time before might have accepted the situation and are willing to accept any device that would enable them to perform desired task. However, some with long period of vision loss may have adapted to their impaired vision status and may therefore, not be motivated to try low vision devices.

Knowledge of the assistance that the patient has previously received is also important. This will include any previous eye and low vision examinations and whatever prescriptions given by the previous professional. It is important to know level of motivation of the patient regarding low vision devices. In general, advantages, disadvantages and limitations of possible devices may briefly be discussed. A highly motivated patient, especially one who has a purpose for which they he or she is seeking low vision devices, will be ready to try the devices to improve his or her vision.

There is no hard and fast rule for effective case history taking as it is a dynamic process. While there is no standard format, the practitioner must learn to initiate and maintain a steady flow of communication during the case history.

Generally, the case history may proceed as follows:

The Chief Complaint

What is the main reason why you are visiting today? Or how can I be of assistance to you today? The chief complaint is important because it helps the practitioner to know the main concern of the patient and what he or she should pay attention to in terms of the visual examination and prescription. This is particularly important in low vision care because the practitioner must focus on a specific goal of the patient, if he or she is to succeed in helping the patient. The exact visual need of the patient must be clearly established. Specific needs and motivation of the patient should be ascertained because low vision devices are not meant for many tasks but each is for limited specific tasks, especially if the working distances differ. Where the patient needs to perform more than one task at different distances, different devices may have to be prescribed. When the patient has stated his or her chief complaint, the next question can be: Are there any other problems? In most cases, the patient has a secondary task that he or she wants to perform.

Ocular History

What is the cause or what have you been told is the cause of your vision loss?

Do you think the vision problem is stable or deteriorating?

Is it slow or fast in deterioration?

A stable vision is desirable, as a deteriorating vision will require regular changing of the visual devices due to power variation.

When was the last eye examination that you have had? Who was the examiner? What was the diagnosis? What was prescribed? Is what was prescribed still being used? If no, why?

Visual Capability

Do you recognize people by face? Do you have difficulty with location of objects placed at any particular side: up, down, right or left? Do you watch television? If so, at what distance? Do you read or write? At what distance? Do you read large or normal print? Do you read magazines? Do you see better when you adjust your head to any particular side? Do you crash into objects or do you find it difficult locating objects when in a particular part of the room? Do you step on things or do you often hit your head against objects?

Mobility

Do you walk independently indoors, outdoors, or in strange places? Do you occasionally or usually use a cane to move around indoors or outdoors? Do you go out or travel without a companion? Do you drive? Do you experience problem climbing a step?

Educational Status or History

What is your level of education? Did you attend regular school or school for the visually impaired? Did you use Braille or large print for your study? Do you currently use normal print, large print or Braille? What is your future aspiration in terms of education (*for young patients*)?

Occupation

Are you currently working? If so, which work do you do? What are your major occupational activities? Have you changed your work due to your eye problem? (If yes)Which work did you before the eye problem?

Hobbies

What are your current hobbies? What other hobbies would you like to engage in? Have you changed your hobbies because of your eye problems? What were your hobbies before your eye problem?

Optical Devices

Have you heard of low vision optical devices? If yes, have you used or tried any optical devices before? Do you currently use an optical device? If yes, what device have you tried or used and for what purpose? Who prescribed the device for you? Where did you obtain it? Is the device useful to you?

Medical History

When last did you undergo a medical examination, and for what reason? Who is your doctor?

Are you presently on any medication? What is the medication for?

Have you had any accident with head or eye injury requiring medical or surgical intervention in the past?

Do you have any systemic disease such as diabetes or hypertension? If yes, are you receiving treatment?

Illumination

Do you see clearer in the day or in the night? Do you use sunglasses? If so, why?

Are you sensitive to light? Does room light make you uncomfortable? Do you use visors or hats to reduce overhead light? Do you prefer high, medium or low level of illumination? Do you find it difficult adjusting when you go from light into dark and vice versa?

Family Ocular and Systemic History

Does any member of your family have vision or eye problems such as cataract, glaucoma or macular degeneration? Has any member of your family had eye surgery? If so, for what purpose? Does any member of your family have systemic problems such as diabetes or hypertension?

The above method of taking case history is simply a guide for the procedure. The trend of the history will vary significantly according to the patient being dealt with and his or her responses.

Following the case history, the tests that may need to be conducted are briefly described below. Detailed procedures will not be presented because they are similar to those for the normally sighted patients. Differences, where necessary, will be stated.

External and internal eye examination

Using the penlight, ophthalmoscope and the slit lamp, the lid margin, cornea and conjunctiva can be examined for scars or signs of diseases. The ophthalmoscope (preferably with dilated pupil, if possible) and slit lamp can be used for the examination of the internal part of the eye. The purpose of these tests is to establish the cause of the low vision or any other ocular pathology.

The procedures may also help to establish whether the eye condition is active or not. Tissues or structures to be examined will include the cornea, anterior chamber, iris, crystalline lens, vitreous humour, and the fundus (macular, optic nerve head as well as other parts of the retina).

Visual Acuity Measurement

Visual acuity values are very important in low vision care as they are used to determine whether or not the low vision patient qualifies for certain benefits, sports, and occupations. The values are also used to monitor the progress of eye diseases. If the disease is progressive, it may decrease the value of the visual acuity and if there is improvement in the eye condition, may improve visual acuity. Most importantly, acuity values are used in calculating the power of magnifying devices required by a low vision patient. The visual acuity values to be measured for a low vision patient include the distance and near (intermediate visual acuity may be measured, if considered necessary). The acuities are to be measured with and without current prescriptions of the patient. If considered necessary, in order to encourage the patient, it is recommended that the visual acuity be measured first with the current glasses, if available.

Distance Visual Acuity Charts

A variety of charts are available for evaluating visual acuity at far. Charts with isolated or grouped letters or numerals are useful. The distance Snellen acuity charts used in the routine clinical procedures are not recommended for low vision evaluation because there are no letters beyond 6/60 (20/200) (1.0 logMAR) and many low vision patients have poorer vision than this can measure. A low vision chart should have acuity rows, which can measure acuity up to 6/360 (20/1200) with intermediate gradations than is found in the Snellen acuity charts[1]. Several charts have been designed specifically for measuring visual acuity for the partially sighted and are commercially available. A common example is the Feinbloom chart, a few pages of which are shown in figures below.

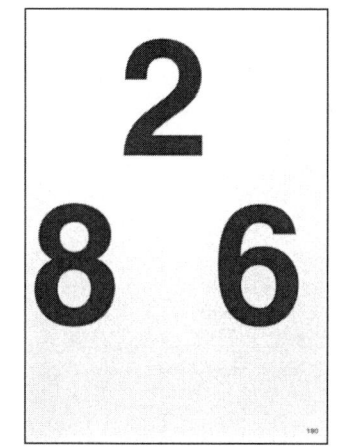

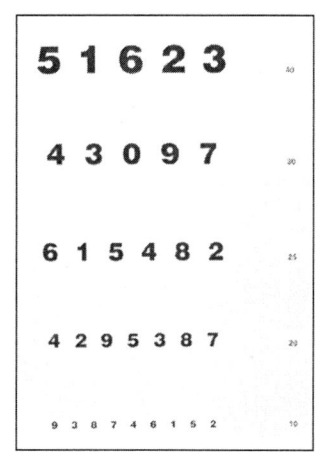

Figures 3: Photos of a few pages of the Feinbloom distance acuity.

Another chart for acuity measurement for visually impaired patients is the logarithm of Minimum Angle of Resolution (logMAR) chart designed by Bailey and Lovie or any of its variations[2]. There are several practical advantages of the use of the Bailey-Lovie chart or its variations and the logMAR visual acuity notation. According to the designers, they offer both flexibility and precision in the measurement of acuity in the moderately or severely impaired patients leading to the prediction of magnification needs. Also, they afford the ability to measure and score low acuity values accurately. Another advantage of the logMAR charts is the ease of conversion to standard test distance values when non-standard test distances are employed in the measurement of the VA. An example of a logMAR chart[3] is shown in figure 3.0. The Snellen, and logMAR equivalents are shown in Table 3.1.

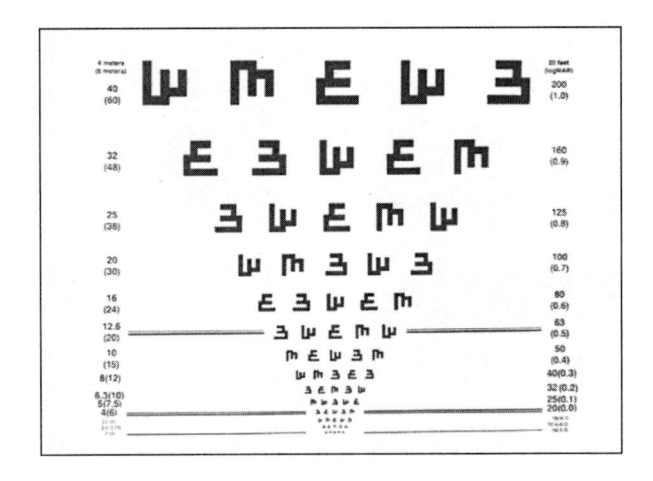

Figure 3.0: Photo of a logMAR distance visual acuity chart for illiterate and young children.

(Oduntan & Briggs Chart, 1999).

Letter size	Snellen Acuity 20 feet	Snellen Acuity 6 meters	MAR	LogMAR
87.3	20/200	6/60	10.0	1.0
69.4	20/160	6/48	8.0	0.9
55.1	20/130	6/38	6.3	0.8
43.8	20/100	6/30	5.0	0.7
34.8	20/80	6/24	4.0	0.6
27.6	20/60	6/18	3.0	0.5
21.9	20/50	6/15	2.5	0.4
17.4	20/40	6/12	2.0	0.3
13.8	20/30	6/10	1.7	0.2
11.9	20/25	6/8	1.3	0.1
8.7	20/20	6/6	1.0	0.0
6.9	20/15	6/5	0.8	-0.1
5.5	20/15	6/4	0.7	-0.2
4.4	20/10	6/3	0.5	-0.3

Table 3.1: Showing acuity letter sizes (millimetres) and the relationships between the Snellen 20 feet, Snellen 6 meters and LogMAR acuities. MAR is minimum angle of resolution. The Snellen acuities are in ratios of 1.2589 while the logMAR rows are in ratios of 0.1 logMAR.

Quite often, the visual acuity of a patient is poorer than can be measured at 6 m (20 ft), so that it becomes necessary to reduce the testing distance. According to Bailey and Lovie, a logMAR chart facilitates this process because for each 0.1 log unit reduction in viewing distance, there is a 0.1 log unit increase in the angular subtense of all the letters in every row of the chart, therefore resulting in one line improvement in visual acuity. In order to facilitate this conversion to the standard testing distance of 6 meters, the testing distance must be reduced by dividing by a ratio of 0.1 log unit (step) or 0.12589. The testing distance will then be (4.8, 3.8, 3.0…meters) or (16, 12.5, 10.8… feet) depending on which notation is used. The visual acuity can then be adjusted to the standard distance, because for every unit decrease in visual acuity, there will be a corresponding improvement in visual acuity. Example: Suppose a patient was tested at a reduced distance of 3 meters, and he or she could read the 6/30 letter, his or her acuity should be recorded as 3/30. As the testing distance was reduced by three logMAR steps, the six meter acuity values will be 3 steps higher up on the chart, which will be 6/60 (20/200) (1.0 logMAR).

Measuring and Scoring

Visual acuity should be measured monocularly and binocularly. Where there is an existing pair of spectacles, the powers should be verified and visual acuity measured with them. The measurement should be started with the largest visual acuity letters. Preferably, the measurement should also be done at 3 meters (10 feet) with the Feinbloom acuity chart or a similar chart. Further, in order to encourage the patient, the better eye should be tested first. The best line that the patient can read should be established. If necessary, longer or shorter test distances can then be used. The routine procedure for measurement of visual acuity should be employed. The patient should be allowed, but not forced, to guess at threshold. The subject is also encouraged to read until all letters on a row are missed. The logMAR scoring system uses an interpolated method where, in a chart with 5 letters per row, each letter read or missed is scored a value of 0.02 logMAR. For example, suppose on a standard chart (**Figure 4.2**), a patient read the two top rows (1.0 and 0.9) and two letters in the 0.8 logMAR row, the best row read (0.9) should be noted, and the logMAR values (2 x 0.02 = 0.4) of the 2 letters that were read in the lower row should be subtracted from the logMAR value of the best line (0.9 -0.04 = 0.86). The acuity value for the patient logMAR) may then be recorded as 0.86 logMAR.

In clinical practice, visual acuity may be scored as counting finger (CF) at a specified distance when a patient cannot read optotypes on a standard chart. For low vision patients, however, it is not advisable to record visual acuity as finger counting because such value may not allow the practitioner to calculate the power of the magnifier required by the patient. Quantitatively, this has been estimated by the World Health Organization (WHO)[4] to be equivalent to 1/60 or (6/360) 20/1200. This quantitative value is useful in predicting the magnification of the visual device to be prescribed for the patient. For practical purposes therefore, counting fingers can be recorded as 1/60 (6/360) or

20/1200. This can then be useful in estimating the magnification that may be required by the patient.

Near Visual Acuity Measurement

A common presenting goal of low vision patients is to be able to perform near tasks such as reading. Near visual acuity values have been recommended for calculating magnifying powers of devices needed by low vision patients for near tasks. Printed material presents a more complex and congested task than does acuity letters; there is often poor agreement between reading acuity and distance letter acuity and these discrepancies become most pronounced when there is a disturbance of macular function as in macular degeneration and amblyopia.

There are several near acuity charts which are commercially available for visual acuity measurement. They include those with isolated letters, grouped letters or numerals (two or more letters or numerals), and paragraphs (Figures 3.1 – 3.3). A numeral chart arranged by Dr Feinbloom (Figure 3.1) has single, double and triple numerals in 24, 18, 14, 10, 7, 5, and 4 point. This type of chart is useful for children and adults, especially those who are able to read numerals but not alphabet or words.

Alphabet charts especially those designed with the logMAR method (Figure 3.2) are useful for near acuity measurement for low vision patients. As the most common goal of low vision patients is reading (usually continuous prints), it is advisable that visual acuity be evaluated with charts designed with words (Figure 4.3) or continuous prints, preferably designed according to the logMAR principles (logarithmic progression). Such charts include the Bailey and Lovie near reading chart (Figure 4.4, below) (obtainable from the National Research Institute of Australia). Another useful chart is the MNREAD chart (obtainable from the Light House, New York).

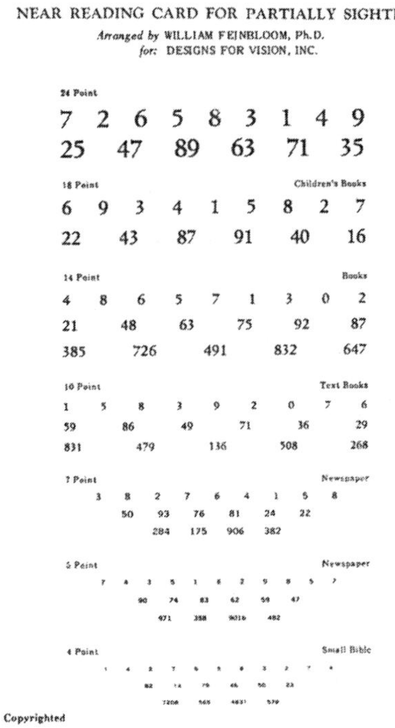

NEAR READING CARD FOR PARTIALLY SIGHTED
Arranged by WILLIAM FEINBLOOM, Ph.D.
for: DESIGNS FOR VISION, INC.

24 Point

7 2 6 5 8 3 1 4 9
25   47   89   63   71   35

18 Point   Children's Books

6 9 3 4 1 5 8 2 7
22   43   87   91   40   16

14 Point   Books

4 8 6 5 7 1 3 0 2
21   48   63   75   92   87
385   726   491   832   647

10 Point   Text Books

1 5 8 3 9 2 0 7 6
59   86   49   71   36   29
831   479   136   508   268

7 Point   Newspaper

3 8 2 7 6 4 1 5 8
50   93   76   81   24   22
284   175   906   382

5 Point   Newspaper

7 4 3 5 1 8 2 9 8 2
90   74   83   62   58   47
471   358   9036   482

4 Point   Small Bible

Copyrighted

Figure 3.1: Near reading chart for partially sighted arranged by William Feinbloom for design for vision. *Courtesy of Design for vision, Inc.*

LogMAR Near Charts for Acuity Measurement

Although, Snellen acuity charts are still used by clinicians for examination of both normally sighted and visually impaired patients, the use of logMAR charts are preferable. The advantages of these charts over the Snellen ones for routing clinical and research work have been discussed by several authors. The use of logMAR acuity (word reading or continuous sentences), offer greater advantages for examination and prescription of optical devices for low vision patients.

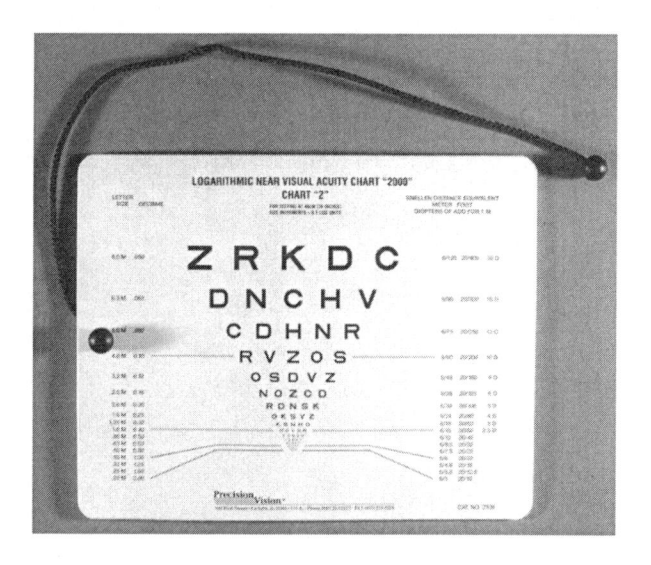

Figure 3.2: Near logMAR alphabet chart (Permission, Precision vision)

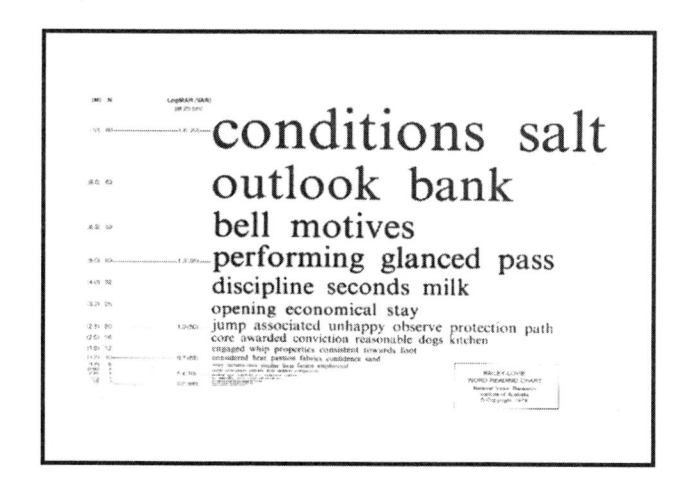

Figure 3.3: Photo of Bailey and Lovie word reading chart (Permission, Precision Vision)

During the near acuity examination of a low vision patient, it is often necessary to reduce the viewing distance to enable the patient to read certain print size on the chart. In this situation, the line to be read at the standard viewing distance of 40 cm, may be presented to the patient at a reduced distance such as 20 cm. Subsequently, the VA value may need to be converted to standard viewing distance (40 cm) value. If a logMAR chart is used for the acuity measurement, the conversion is quite simple, provided that appropriate reduction in viewing distance in steps of 1.2589 is employed. The ease of conversion of the non-standard VA values to standard value is an important feature of the logMAR principle. The process, however, involves series of multiplication and division of viewing distances by logMAR ratio of 1.2589.

For example, a patient could read 0.7 logMAR 5M at a reduced distance of 20 cm. What is the equivalent value of this acuity value at the standard viewing distance of 40cm? By dividing 40 cm by 1.2589 three times, you would arrive at 20 cm. This shows that the viewing distance has been reduced by a factor of 3 logMAR steps. Therefore, the visual acuity at standard viewing distance will be three logMAR steps larger print. This can be calculated by adding 0.3 to 0.7 logMAR 1.0 (10M).

Bailey and Lovie[2] presented another major feature of the logMAR near charts in relation to low vision care: the quantities involved in the optical prescriptions for near vision are proportional to one another. The angular subtense of a print is inversely proportional to the viewing distance, and the dioptric power of the near addition is inversely proportional to the focal distance of the lens. Also, the magnification provided by a device is directly proportional to the dioptric power of the lens, and the threshold print size is inversely proportional to the magnification used or directly proportional to the viewing distance, and so on. The logMAR reading charts can be used to predict optical needs and performance of a patient with an optical device of known power because of these features. Powers and focal lengths of magnifiers are particularly important in low vision care, because magnifying lenses are high power plus lenses, consequently, their foci are very important because, if the patient does not look through these, clear vision will not be enjoyed.

The use of logMAR chart facilitates calculation of focal points for optical devices. For example, If a patient, who previously used a 2x magnifier (+8.00D), has the power of his prescription increased to 5x (+20.00D). From 8 to 20 is four steps upward shift in the 1.2589 logMAR scale. The focal length (viewing distance) will also change (reduce) by four logMAR steps from 12.5cm to 5cm. This implies that, if the dioptric power of the magnifier required by the patient is increased by a certain logMAR ratio, the viewing distance (focal distance of the lens) will need to be reduced by the same ratio for the patient to see the print in focus, which will obviously increase dioptric demand. Direct proportionality of the magnification with dioptric power is important in low vision care because, as dioptric power is increased, it may be necessary to know the magnification provided. Another example: If a patient has a magnifier which provided magnification of 2x and it is anticipated that, due to change in visual need, the patient will now benefit from a magnification of 4x. The magnification has changed by logMAR ratio factor of 3; therefore the dioptric power of the device will need to be changed by a logMAR ratio of 3 steps from +8.00D to +16.00D. Therefore, if the ratio of increase in magnification required is known, the dioptric power needed will just be an increase in ratio of the original dioptric power. Similarly, the working distance will change by the same ratio from 12.5 to 6.25 cm.

The logMAR principles can also be used to predict the print size that a patient is expected to read when the dioptric power of the magnifier changes. For example, if a patient can read logMAR 0.6 (4M) at 40 cm with a magnifier power of +5.00D. If the power is increased to +8.00 D, what print size is the patient expected to read? The change in power is 2 steps increase on the logMAR scale. The patient will therefore, be expected to read 2 steps down the logMAR chart, which is equivalent to 0.4 logMAR. Similarly, the power of the magnifier needed by a patient to read a particular print can be estimated by calculating ratio of decrease in print size. The direct proportionality of print size and viewing distance using the logMAR chart can be explained as follows: As the viewing distance is reduced, the angular subtense of the print increases correspondingly, therefore the patient will be expected to read smaller print size that corresponds to the number of logMAR steps that the viewing distance has been reduced as shown in the following example. A patient can read 6.3M (0.9 logMAR) (N51) at 25 cm. If it is anticipated that the patient will achieve her visual goal if she is able to read 2M (0.3 logMAR) (N16) print size at the same distance, which is 5 logMAR steps decrease in print size; decreasing the viewing distance by a factor of 5 logMAR steps from 25 cm to 8 cm will afford the visual resolution needed by the patient to read the print.

Illumination level is an important factor in the measurement of visual acuity for low vision patients because, with variation of illumination, there may be a significant improvement or reduction in visual acuity. While increased illumination will lead to an improvement in visual acuity in certain patients such as those with macular degeneration, it may lead to deterioration in others such as those with albinism or aniridia. The visual acuity should, therefore, be measured with different levels of illumination (low, medium and high), and the level that improves the acuity recorded.

Contrast Sensitivity

Contrast sensitivity may be reduced in most low vision patients especially those with conditions such as diabetic retinopathy or macular degeneration. Patients with reduced contrast sensitivity may have problems in performing activities of daily living because of the variation in contrast from one object to another. It is, therefore, important to measure contrast sensitivity for low vision patients in order to assess the problems that they may be experiencing in the real world. In addition, it has been established that contrast sensitivity measured at low to mid-spatial frequencies is a useful predictor of reading rates in partially sighted adults[5,6]. The Vistech contrast sensitivity chart may be used, but in view of reading performance evaluation, however, the Pelli-Robson chart[7] has been recommended for assessment of contrast sensitivity for low vision patients because it measures contrast sensitivity at the spatial frequencies shown to be predictive of reading rate. This factor makes the Pelli-Robson chart superior to other contrast sensitivity charts for low vision evaluation.

Colour Vision Test

Many conditions of the visual system such as diabetic retinopathy, macular degeneration and optic atrophy may be associated with colour vision defects. The importance of the colour vision testing is thus, to enable the practitioner determine the colour discrimination status, which may provide information on the visual function of the patient. Colour deficiency may be an indication of cone dysfunction, therefore, may be associated with poor visual acuity. For instance, typical (rod) monochromats have no functioning cone receptors and is associated with poor visual acuity, 6/30 or worse, photophobia and nystagmus[8]. It is therefore, advised that colour vision perception be evaluated in addition to visual acuity when the latter is poor.

A simple test that can be administered and scored quickly is the Farnsworth panel D15. (See Figure 3.6A below.). This test is a shortened version of the Farnsworth-Munsell 100 Hue test. There are two test types: saturated (standard test) and desaturated. The desaturated type is more demanding because the colour samples are less saturated and are lighter (by three units of Munsell value) than the standard type. Each of the tests consists of a set of 15 colour caps (Figure 3.6B) and scoring sheets. Under the caps are numbers (1-15) which can be used to check the correct order or otherwise of the caps (Figure 3.4). The colour caps are to be randomly organized by the examiner, and the patient is expected to arrange them in proper order according to their changing hues with regard to the reference cap, P. When the patient has arranged the caps, the box is closed and turned upside down to check the order of arrangement of the caps (Figure 3.5). The result is to be plotted on a score sheet (Figure 3.5) by linking the numbers 1-15 for a subject with normal colour vision. A subject with deficient colour vision will mix the numbers. The plotted errors will dictate the type of colour vision deficiency.

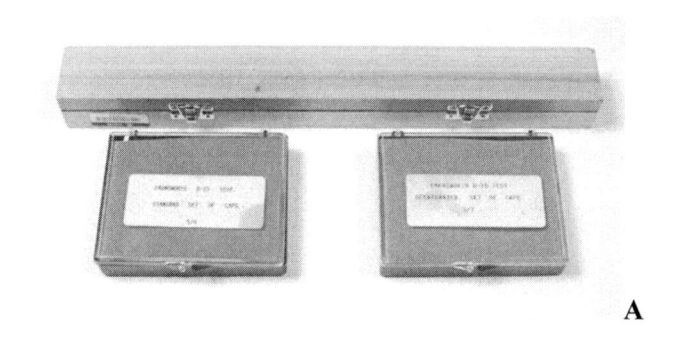

A

Figure 3.4:

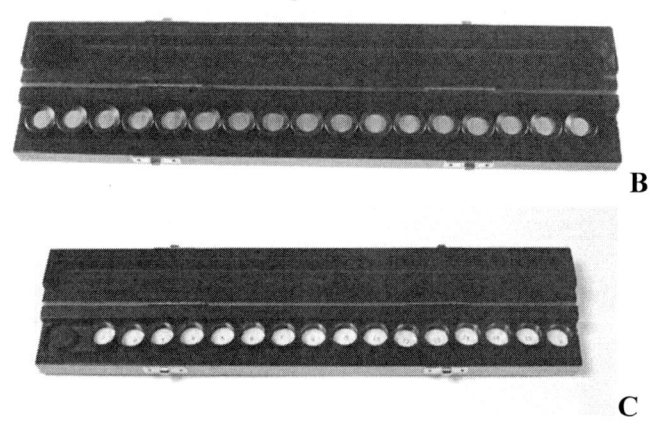

B

C

Figure 3.5:

Farnsworth panel D-15: **A.** Wooden box in which the caps are arranged and the plastic containers of the saturated (left) and unsaturated (right) colour caps.

B. Arrangement of the caps in correct order. **C.** Numbers showing the order of the caps arrangement.

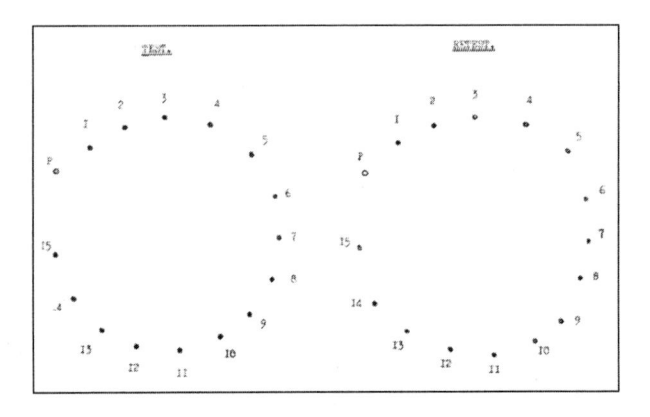

Figure 3.6: Score sheet for Farnsworth panel D-15, saturated and unsaturated tests.

Visual Fields

Patients with reduced peripheral visual field face serious mobility problems as they tend to bump into objects and frequently fall. Those with central field loss have difficulty with reading at near or other near tasks. The extent of the visual field loss and the density of the scotoma areas are very informative in low vision care, since the density and location of the visual field will be useful in explaining the visual difficulties that the patient experiences, the visual field often correlated with the visual difficulties that the patient experiences. Goldman perimeter, Tangent screen and Amsler grid are very useful tests for most cases of low vision.

Peripheral Field Assessment

In a variety of clinical situations, static perimetry have been found to be superior to kinetic perimetry for low vision cases such as age-related macular degeneration[9,10]. The Goldmann Perimeter especially is a useful field charting test in cases of glaucoma and neurological problems resulting in field defects and should be used where considered possible.

Central Field Assessment

The tangent screen is useful for evaluating the integrity of the central 30 degrees of the visual field. In cases of poor vision due to central scotoma, the patient may experience difficulty seeing the test target and the fixation target. A large enough target that the patient can see should thus be used as the fixation target. A large cross drawn with a chalk with the centre at the position of the fixation target can also be used, if there is a problem with target fixation. The patient will be instructed to fixate where the vertical and horizontal lines of the cross appear to intersect.

The Amsler grid chart consisting of a grid of horizontal and vertical lines, is used to examine the central 10 degrees of visual field surrounding fixation point[11]. It is a simple test that enables the examiner to evaluate the visual problems associated with the beginning and other stages of various macular problems such as age-related macular degeneration or macular hole. Amsler grid test has been found to be very useful in cases of comprised macular integrity, as it is able to reveal slight defects in some pre-age-related macular degeneration patients[12]. It is particularly useful to monitor stages of central field loss in low vision patients, therefore, should be performed alongside other visual field tests.

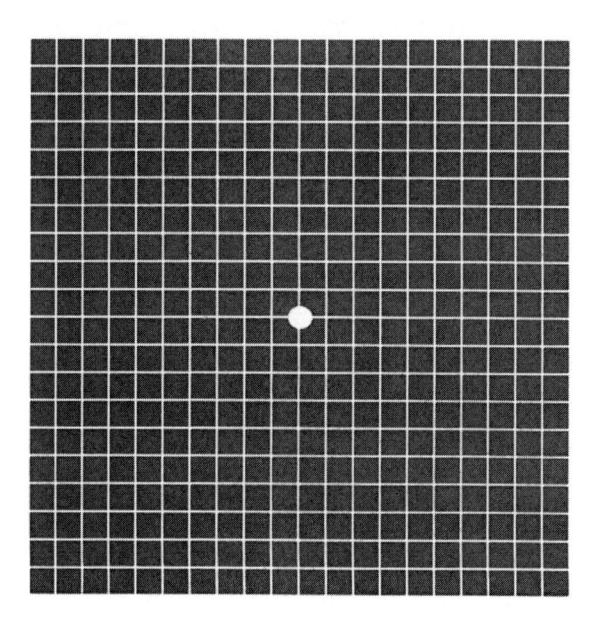

Figure 3.7 A: Amsler grid used for testing macular integrity.

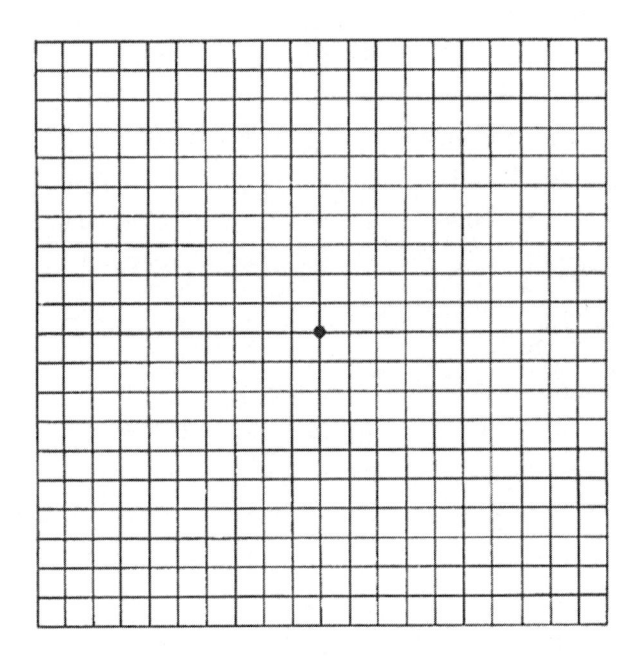

Figure 3.7B: Recording sheet for Amsler grid findings.

Retinoscopy and Keratometry

Objective tests such as retinoscopy and keratometry are not quite as reliable as subjective refraction for examining low vision patients. They, however, help to provide some crude values that can be used as starting point for the subjective refraction.

Retinoscopy

The procedure for the static retinoscopy is similar to that done on normally-sighted persons, but there are cases where poor reflex will dictate the need for radical retinoscopy (working at a shorter test distance and perhaps, off axis, that allows reflex to be seen)[1]. Retinoscopic values may be unreliable in cases of cloudy media. Trial lenses and trial frames are preferable to phoropter in performing retinoscopy for low vision patients because they enable the patient to orientate his or her head as desired by the examiner. Also, lenses can be changed in higher lens powers as necessary.

Keratometry

Keratometric values are quite useful in cases where high astigmatism or irregular anterior corneal surfaces contributes to poor vision as in keratoconus. The procedure is similar to that employed for normally sighted person. The keratometric values may be useful in determining the amount of astigmatism due to the anterior corneal surface.

Subjective Refraction

Subjective refraction is a useful test in low vision patient examination. Even where no useful value is obtained from the objective test such as retinoscopy, the subjective may become the only test to be relied upon for refractive correction and subsequent prescription of optical device power. An accurate subjective refraction should be performed with a trial frame rather than a phoropter, to allow the patient a wide field of view and permit eccentric viewing, when necessary[13]. Also, as with the retinoscopy, trial frame are preferable as they permits rapid lens power changes such as ±2.00D ±3.00D or ±5.00D[1]. The subjective sight testing may commence with whatever available retinoscopic values. If a previous pair of glasses is available and the powers of the lenses are considered to be more reliable than the retinoscopic values, then these can be used as starting point for the subjective refraction. As with the normally sighted patients, the spherical errors have to be neutralized first. If the poor vision is suspected to be due to high refractive errors, lens changes may be in steps as high as ± 3.00 D spheres if considered necessary, depending on the degree of the suspected refractive error. The steps can then be decreased to ±2.00 D and refined with ±1.00 D or ±0.50 D. The visual acuity chart must be placed at a reasonably reduced distance (three, two or one meter if necessary). The distance may be increased as the vision improves. The lenses are changed until the best sphere is obtained.

Following the determination of the best spherical lens/es, the astigmatic component of the refractive error can then be neutralized. If refractive cylinder is suspected to be high, for the patient to observe differences in the Jackson cross cylinder powers, a ±1.00 DC or ±2.00 DC cross cylinder may be used rather than ± 0.50DC or ±0.25 DC. Subsequently, smaller power e.g. ± 0.5 may be used. The value of a starting correcting cylinder can also be that obtained from the retinoscopic value or from the powers of an existing spectacle. The axis and power of the best correcting cylinder should be determined in the usual manner and visual acuity measured. The refractive power findings (objective and subjective) with the corresponding visual acuity values should be recorded.

It is not advisable to prescribe distance spectacles for a low vision patient, except there is a significant improvement in visual acuity of at least one or more acuity lines. If the visual acuity values in both eyes are similar or have a difference of less than one acuity line, the patient may benefit from binocular devices. Therefore, binocular vision assessment should be carried out. If the patient is a presbyope, a tentative reading addition should be determined using any appropriate method.

Binocular Vision

Binocular vision assessment is not usually performed for low vision patients because, in most cases, the acuity values and corrective powers in both eye differ significantly. However, in spite of poor vision, certain low vision patients may benefit from binocular vision assessment. Binocular vision anomaly may contribute to the ocular symptoms experienced by some low vision patients. A low vision patient may also have to use binocular devices, which may precipitate binocular symptoms. Therefore, it is important to have an idea of the binocular vision status of low vision patient where evaluation is possible. It is important to note that certain systemic and ocular disorders can induce binocular problems. For example, apart from visual acuity, visual field and contrast sensitivity loss, other functional deficits of vision may occur due to diabetes. Cranial nerve palsies (III, IV and VI) causing extra-ocular muscle paresis, resulting in diplopia are not uncommon in patients with diabetes[14]. Since both ocular pathology and binocular anomaly may induce near vision problems which may affect visual function at near, it is important to measure binocular function at near so that associated problems can be taken care of independently. Whether or not the patient will be using a binocular assistive device/s, the binocular vision status should be assessed using simple methods such as the cover tests, worth's 4 dots, vergence, and eye movement tests, where possible. Where possible, elimination of binocular vision anomaly will enhance visual comfort and facilitate training in the use of low vision devices.

Evaluation of Appropriate Level of Illumination

Determination of appropriate level of illumination is an important part of the subjective examination of a low vision patient. The effects of various levels of illumination (high, medium and low) on the improvement of visual acuity with the subjective refractive powers (distance and near) should be evaluated. The illuminance level that provides the best visual acuity values should be recorded. This will subsequently be a part of the information to be provided to the patient for effective use of the prescribed devices.

References

Mehr B.E and Freid, AN. Low vision care. Professional Press. USA, Chicago, 1975.

Bailey IL & Lovie JE. New design principle for acuity letter chart. Am J Optom Physiol Opt. 1976; 53: 740-745.

Oduntan AO and Briggs ST. An Arabic letter distance VA chart for young children and illiterate adults. Ophthal Physiol Opt. 1999; 19: 431-437.

World Health Organization. International classification of impairment, disabilities and handicaps: A manual of relationship to the consequences of diseases. Geneva. 1980.

Rubin GS & Legge GE. Psychophysics of reading. VI – the role of contrast in low vision. Vision Res. 1989; 29: 89-91.

Leat SJ and Woodhouse JM. Reading performance with low vision aids: relationship with contrast sensitivity. Ophthal Physiol Opt. 1993; 13: 9-16.

Pelli DG & Robson JG. The design of a new letter for measuring contrast sensitivity. Clin Vis Sci. 1988; 2:187-199.

Birch J. Color deficiency: An introduction. Optician. 1999; 218: 22-25.

Fortney GL and Krohn MA. The limitations of kinetic perimetry in early scotoma detection. Ophthalmol. 1978; 85: 287-293.

Yellen M & Sherman J. Static vs. dynamic visual field evaluation, with emphasis on the utility of the Friedmann visual field analyzer. J Am Optom Assoc. 1979; 50: 95-99.

Amsler M. Earliest symptom of diseases of the macular. Brit J Ophthalmol. 1953, 37: 521-537.

Swann PG, Lovie-Kitchin JE. Age-related maculopathy. II: The nature of the central visual field loss. Ophthal Physiol Opt. 1991; 11:59-70.

Bailey IL. Refracting low vision patients. Optom monthly. 1978; 69: 131-134.

Cooke JB, Cockrane AL. A practical guide to low vision management of patients with diabetes. Clin Exp Optom. 2001; 84:155-161.

Bibliography

Brower J. A practical guide to low vision assessment and dispensing. Optom today. 2001; Feb. 9: 34-36.

Brown B, Reading performance in low vision patients: relation to contrast and contrast sensitivity. Am J Optom Physiol Opt. 1981; 8: 218-226.

Eperjesi F, Fowler, CW, Evans BJ. Effects of filters on reading speed in normal and low vision due to age-related macular degeneration. Ophthal. Physiol Optics. 2004; 24: 17-25.

Johnston AW. Making sense of M, N and logMAR systems of specifying visual acuity. Problems in Optom. 1991; 3: 394-407.

Leat S and Rumney N. A simplified approach to low vision assessment. 1. Optician. 1990; Sep 14 :11-19.

Lovie-Kitchin JE, Whittaker SG. Prescribing near magnification for low vision patients. Clin Exp Optom. 1999: 82: 214-224.

Oduntan AO. Visual acuity measurement for statistical analysis and graphical representation. S Afr Optom. 2001; 60: 97-101.

Rundstrom MM, Eperjesi F. Is there a need for binocular evaluation in low vision? Ophthal Physiol Opt. 1995; 15: 525-528.

Strong G, Woo G. A distance visual acuity chart incorporating some new design features. Arch. Ophthalmol 1985; 103: 44-46.

Chapter 4
Clinical Assessment of Children With Low Vision

Vision requirements for children are not the same as for adults, therefore one cannot directly apply the results from adults to children[1]. For assessment of children with low vison, children-oriented test charts for visual acuity and contrast sensitivity should be available. Functional assistive materials such as thick line papers and crayons, or thick nib pens should be available in the clinic room as well. Pre-assessment visit by the child and parents may be necessary to enable the child to get familiarized with the clinic environment and the parents to have a relevant discussion with the practitioner regarding what they should bring on the day of the assessment. Although, the assessment of visually impaired children is broadly similar to that of adults, there are a few differences in the approach employed. Many of the tests would require a flexible approach, and will include both formal and informal assessment. Also, it is important to assess how the child uses his or her residual vision[2].

Observation

Careful observation of the child is important during the pre-assessment and assessment visits. The practitioner should, make a keen observation of the child as he or she is brought to the clinic by the parents, especially how he or she uses the residual vision. Observing the child's posture, eye movements and tracking skills should be noted[3]. The parents and teachers could be involved in the process of gathering information about their observations of how the child uses his or her vision for various activities. Knowledge of how the child uses his or her residual vision at home and at school is important. The parents and teachers could be instructed to observe the child and note all the physical and visual characteristics that they consider as abnormal. Difficulties encountered by the child in the home and school environment should be noted too. Such information should then be passed to the low vision practitioner prior to assessment. A questionnaire regarding the observations and case history may be developed and given to the teacher and parents for completion prior to the assessment exercise.

Case History

The assistance of parents or guardians is important during the case history stage of the visual assessment of the children. The case history can be provided more reliably by the parents or guardians of a pre-school child or infant than the child or somebody else. Even, younger children do not respond well to lengthy questioning. It is, therefore, important to rely on the parents as much as possible for important questions. Where necessary and possible, questions could be directed the child. Parents are, nevertheless, a very useful source of information about a young child. Parents have a more practical understanding of their child's abilities and limitations than can be obtained during conventional clinical assessment[3].

School-age children can contribute effectively to a case history but the history should be child oriented. The parents should be involved in confirming and supplementing the information provided by the child. The parents of a child with congenital visual impairment will be able to provide better information than the child, even when the child is able to express himself or herself. Also, the developmental milestone, medical and ophthalmic history of a child, can only be presented accurately by the parents. A questionnaire covering all the relevant aspects of the case history including on how the child uses his or her residual vision at home may be developed for completion by the parents or guardian prior to assessment. Even here a questionnaire is used to collect information for case history, parents will still be asked questions during the visual assessment.

Visual Acuity (Distance and Near)

Distance and near visual acuity charts that are appropriate for the age and knowledge of the child should be used for acuity assessment. For literate children, LogMAR charts designed for children are recommended, but in the case of children who are not able to read, other appropriate test charts could be used. Acuity charts designed with letters or numerals are not appropriate for infants and young children as they may not be able to perform the task required. In such instances, charts that require the matching of letters such as symbol charts can also be uses. The Lea Hyvarinen chart (Figure 4.1), which has only four symbols (circle, square, house, and heart) is a useful alternative as well. Other appropriate charts are the Sheridan-Gardiner chart (Figure 4.2), the Kay picture (Figure 4.3) test, Lea number chart (4.4) and Stycar tests. For infants, preferential looking or visually evoked potential techniques will provide useful information.

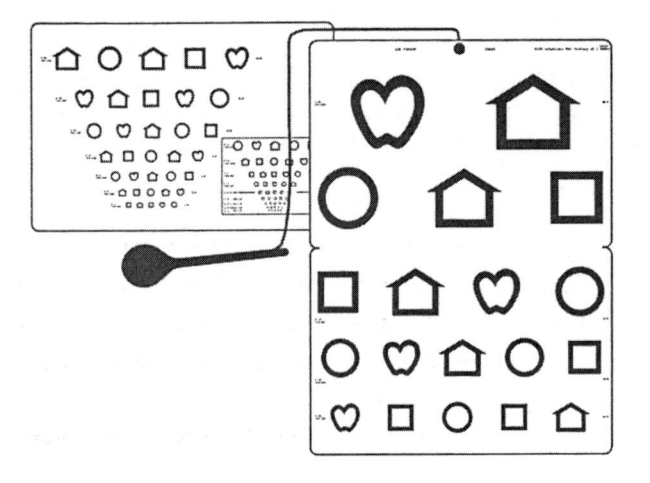

Figure 4.1: Lea Hyvarinen charts for testing infants and young children.

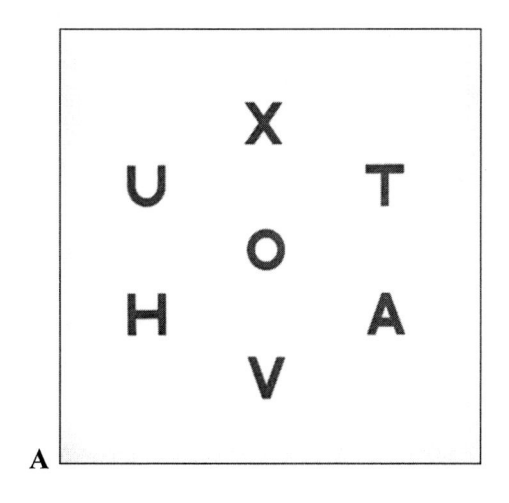

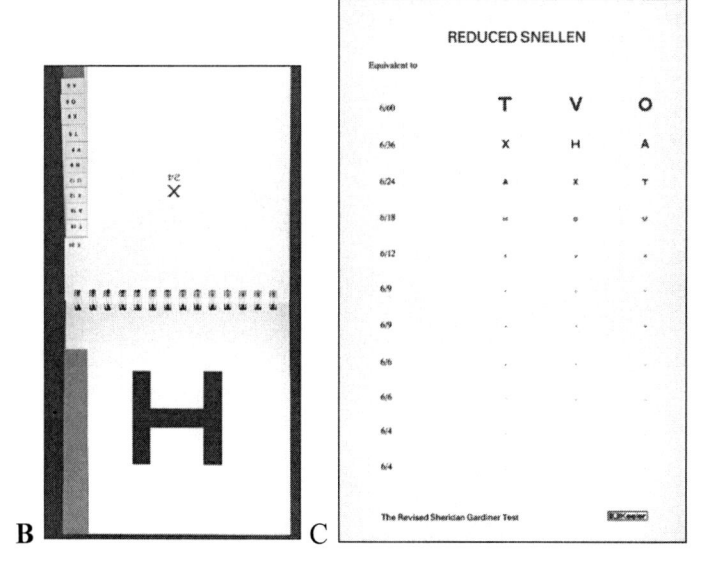

Figure 4.2: The revised Sheridan Gardiner charts for testing visual acuity for young school-age children. Charts A and B for distance vision testing, and C, for near vision testing.

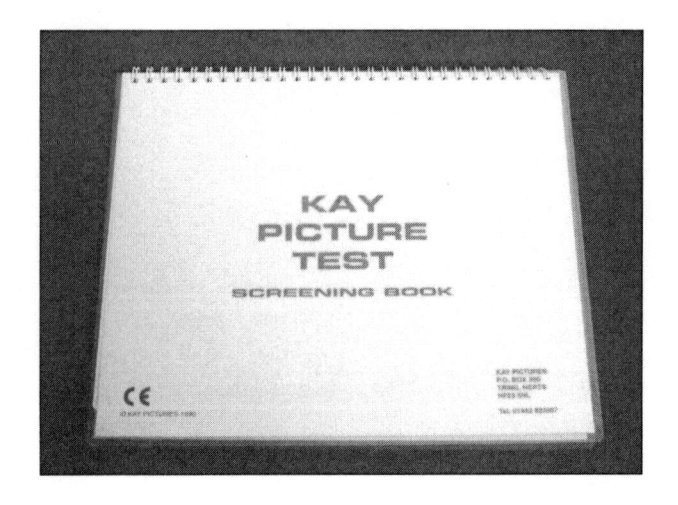

Figure 4.3 A: The Kay picture test for testing young children.

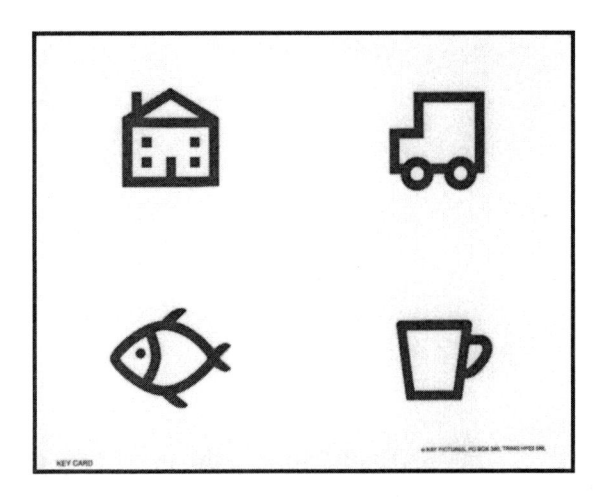

Figure 4.3 B: A page of the Kay Picture test.

Commercially available preferential looking techniques include the Teller and Keeler Acuity cards which use grating stimuli and the Cardiff acuity test which uses picture stimuli to elicit preferential looking. It is often useful to evaluate distance visual acuity by more than one method as this helps to check if there is consistency. Where there is nystagmus, the reading material should be placed towards the null position (where the nystagmus is minimal). It is important when working with severely impaired children to be aware that their poor responses may be a result of their level of cognition rather than visual development[4].

Assessing near acuity with younger children is possible using matching techniques with the Lighthouse M letter chart or shape recognition such as the Lea Hyvarinen near chart (Figure 4.1). Both of these charts use the logMAR design format[5]. For those who can read numbers, the Lea number near chart (Figure 4.4) below is very useful.

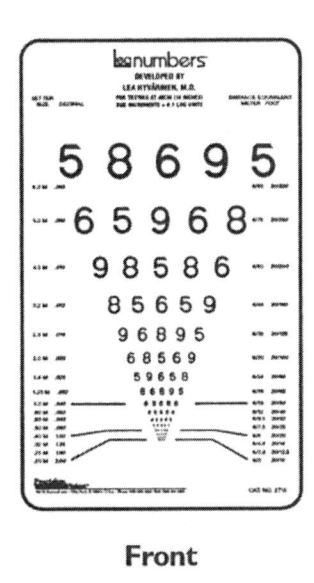

Figure 4.4: Lea numbers visual acuity card.

Retinoscopy and Subjective Refraction

Accurate refraction should be done for all children where possible. The refractive error should be carefully measured and corrected. High refractive errors, especially hyperopia and astigmatism, are common in infants and young children; hence an accurate refraction is important in providing a full visual assessment. For example, many children with albinism have significant refractive errors (spherical and astigmatic), correction of which may result in significant improvement in certain children.

As most children have high accommodation, which may influence refraction, cycloplegic refraction is a necessity in children, particularly as some eye conditions are associated with high refractive errors which need to be neutralized. Following a cycloplegic refraction, further examination may have to be postponed till such time when the effect of cycloplegia has worn off. Near retinoscopy is an important aspect of examination of infants and young children. Where there is horizontal nystagmus, there may be no need to sweep the retinoscope across the pupillary area.

In very young children and infants where subjective refraction is not practicable, objective refraction may be the only choice of refraction. Where subjective refraction is possible, it should be done carefully.

Contrast Sensitivity

Contrast sensitivity provides an evaluation of the visual performance of the child under real life conditions. For children who can read letters, the Bailey and Lovie 10% contrast letters at the reverse side of the standard chart will be useful. Where adult standard type of contrast sensitivity such as the Vistech or Bailey and Lovie contrast charts is not applicable, the Pelli-Robson chart, requiring letter naming can be very useful. The chart, however, requires that the child should be able to read the alphabets. The picture based tests, such as the Hiding-Heidi test (developed by Hyvarinen), which involves comparing cards with high and low contrast targets, may be employed. Others are the Cambridge low contrast grating and the 'Mr Happy' contrast sensitivity charts. These are quite useful for young children who are not able to name letters.

Accommodation

It is necessary to measure amplitude of accommodation in infants and children. Children normally have high accommodation amplitude, which they can use to gain magnification at short working distances. According to Jackson and Sunders[3] preschool children with a visual impairment and normal accommodative response will generally disregard near vision aids, preferring to utilize accommodation and working distances of 5-10cm^3. Children with normal accommodation may naturally hold the page closer than 25cm, and this should be encouraged as it can delay the need for magnifying aids. Holding the print at 8.5cm will utilize 12.00 dioptres of accommodation and give 3x magnification[6] (Magnification = F/4), where F = power of lens). Where there is enough accommodation for this purpose, there may not be a need to prescribe an optical device for near reading.

On the contrary, certain children (especially those with Down's syndrome) are known to have reduced accommodation. It is, therefore, important to have an idea of the amount of accommodation that the child has. It is essential to note that not all children have the high accommodative capability expected for their ages. For school-age children, the standard subjective push up method may be used to estimate the amount of accommodation. For preverbal children, it may be necessary to use a dynamic retinoscopy technique to establish the level of accommodation. When the accommodation possessed cannot support the working distance necessary to provide the magnification required, partial or full power of magnifier may be prescribed.

Visual Field

Estimation of the central and peripheral field is essential for children as well. This may, however, not be easily done on children. When traditional methods of evaluating visual fields are not possible, especially with children less than five years, an estimation of the peripheral field may be attempted by the examiner by positioning himself or herself behind the child and slowly bringing a light source or a small object into the child's field of view from all directions. The point of response to the target is then estimated and recorded[6,7]. For older children, kinetic perimetry using the bowl perimeter or one of the automated perimeters can be used. Confrontation test may be done when considered practicable. The visual field results should be used to advise parents on mobility and posture-related issues[2]. For children, Goldman fields and Humphrey's visual field analyser may be performed binocularly[5].

Keratometry

Where considered necessary and possible, keratometry may be useful in detecting corneal astigmatism in children. The procedure is basically the same as that used in routine examination.

Binocular Vision

Where considered appropriate, binocular function of the child should be assessed using appropriate methods. This will help to avoid binocular vision anomaly symptoms. Reduced convergence or diplopia at near may be difficult for a child to verbalize and may be contributing to difficulties in using low vision devices, particularly if close working distance and high levels of accommodation are used[4].

Colour Vision

The determination of colour vision in children is important as a large proportion of their education is in the form of colour-coded materials. Where possible, colour vision assessment should be done with Farnsworth panel D-15. It has large target sizes and can be used in a matching format to allow use with preschool children[3]. It is, however, not very useful with very young children. Findings of colour vision deficiency and its implications should be discussed with parents and teachers.

References

Al-Abdulkader B, Leat LJ. Reading in children with low vision. J Optom. 2010; 3: 68-74.

Bevan JD. The optometric management of a child with low vision. Aust J Optom. 1983; 66: 142-146.

Jackson AJ and Saunders KJ. The optometric assessment of the visually impaired infant and young child. Ophthal Physiol Opt. 1999; 19: S49-S62.

Jose RT, Smith AJ and Shane KG. Evaluating and stimulating vision in the multiply impaired. J Vis impair blind. 1980; 74: 2-8.

Brower J. A practical guide to low vision assessment and dispensing. Optom today. 2001; Feb. 9: 34-36.

Yellen M and Sherman J. Static vs. dynamic visual field evaluation, with emphasis on the utility of the Friedmann visual field analyzer. J Am Optom Assoc 1979; 50: 95-99.

Bairstow M. Children and low vision. 1999; 218: 16-21.

Bibliography

Bailey IL, Lovie JE. New design principles for visual acuity letter charts. Am J Optom Physiol Opt. 1976; 53: 740-745.

Bailey IL, Lovie JE. The design and use of new near vision chart. Am J Optom Physiol Opt. 1980; 57: 378-387.

Bailey IL. Prescribing low vision reading aids – A new approach. Optom Monthly. 1981.

Faye EE. Clinical Low Vision. 2nd ed. Boston: Little, Brown and Co, 1985.

Fortney GL and Krohn MA. The limitations of kinetic perimetry in early scotoma detection. Ophthalmol. 1978; 85: 287-293.

Stelmack JA, Rosenbloom AA, Brenneman CS, Stelmack TR. Patient's perception of need of low vision devices. J Vis Imp Blind. 2003; 97: 521-516.

Rundstrom MM, Eperjesi F. Is there a need for binocular evaluation in low vision? Ophthal Physiol Opt. 1995; 15: 525-528.

Chapter 5
Principles of Magnification in Low Vision Care

Definition of Magnification with regard to low vision reading at near has generated a lot of controversies in the past. This led to various versions of magnification such as conventional and iso-accommodation magnifications[1], effective magnification[2], apparent magnification[3]. Bailey[4] advocated for discarding the term magnification as a means of quantifying enhancement of visibility of details of near objects. These various terms complicated issues as each meant different term to different authors. According to Bailey[4], apparent magnification was sometimes referred to as angular magnification or perceived magnification, while Relative magnification was sometimes called conventional magnification or effective magnification or traditional magnification or apparent magnification.

Bailey[4] advocated that the term magnification is inappropriate as a means of quantifying vision enhancement at near. The author presented a strong argument in support of his claim that the term magnification is inappropriate and should be discarded. He suggested two terms, namely, Equivalent Viewing Power (EVP) or Equivalent Viewing Distance (EVD) to replace magnification. The term EVD has been subsequently used in an equation to predict power of device needed to enhance reading vision at near. The predictive power can be calculated from the formula[5]:

Required EVD = $\dfrac{\text{Required TPS}}{\text{Current TPS}}$ x Current EVD

Where EVD is the equivalent viewing distance, which is the (closer) distance at which the original object will subtend the same angular size as the angular size of the image formed by the plus spherical lens. Required TPS is threshold print size that the patient wishes to read and current TPS is the current best near acuity of the patient. EVP will be the dioptric power of EVD.

In spite of the strong argument presented by Bailey[4] against the use of the term magnification, and recommendations of possible replacements, the terms EVP and EVD are not popular among low vision care practitioners. The term magnification is as popular as ever. Magnification can simply be defined as an increase in the real size of an object its image size. It is a comparison of a new size to an old size. Magnification is an important concept in low vision care because, a large proportion of assistance that can be rendered to a low vision patient is in the form of magnification of the prints that he or she wants to see or the size of an object that the patient wants to use. It is, therefore, important for a low vision practitioner to understand the principles of magnification in order to be able to provide efficient care for the patient.

A major aspiration of many low vision patients, is to be able to read at near and or far. Reading material at near may be items such as personal letters, books, newspapers or magazines. At far, reading material may be house numbers, bus numbers or sign posts on the road. One of the ways by which a low vision patient can be assisted, is to provide magnification of the print that he or she wants to read. This can be done by increasing the size of the reading material or the object of regard, this enlarges the image size on the retina, thereby providing greater retinal image resolution to the patient. This increase in size or magnification enables the patient to read what he or she wishes to read and was unable to read due to poor vision. Apart from physically increasing the size of the print or object of regard, there are others ways of increasing the size of the retinal image, thereby providing magnification. These various methods will be discussed in this chapter.

i. In low vision care, principles that are often used to achieve magnification include the following:
ii. Increasing the physical size of the object or its image
iii. Moving the object close to the eye
iv. Using various types of magnifiers
v. Using a projector to provide a larger version of the print *et cetera*

Irrespective of which methods employed, the purpose of magnification is to increase the size of the retinal image produced compared to the retinal image size without any device or without reduction of the eye-to-object distance. Magnification can then be defined as the ratio of the enlarged retinal image size to the original retinal image size of the object.

The retinal image of an object is directly proportional to the angle that the image subtends with the eye's exit pupil. Also, the retinal image size of an object is directly proportional to the actual size of the object. The retinal image size of an object can, therefore, be increased by increasing the size of the object, which in turn increases the angle that the object makes with the eye's entrance pupil. Increasing the angular subtense of the object with the eye's entrance pupil subsequently increases the angular subtense of the retinal image at the eye's exit pupil. If the size of an object of regard is increased without changing the distance between the eye and the object, the angular subtense of the object with the eye's entrance pupil is increased, which consequently increases the angular subtense of the retinal image with the eye's exit pupil. Similarly, decreasing the distance between the object of regard and the eye increases the objective angular subtense, which consequently increases the image angular subtense. These ultimately increase the size of the retinal image thereby resulting in greater resolution of the image. No matter which method is used, magnification results from the increase in the angle that the object of regard or its image makes with the eye.

There are 4 types of magnification that are commonly employed in low vision care. These include:

Relative size magnification

i. Relative distance magnification
ii. Angular magnification
iii. Projection magnification

Relative Size Magnification (RSM)

This is the magnification resulting from the increase in the actual size of an object or print that the patient wants to see or use. This type of magnification involves a physical increase in the size of the object of regard or its image. The magnification provided here, is the ratio of the new object (or print) size to the old object (or print) size. Suppose in measuring the visual acuity of a patient, he or she cannot read N8 print, and you decided to try N12 print and the patient is able to read it, the size of the print has been increased (1.5x magnification). It is this increase in size that has provided an increase in resolution, which enables the patient to read the print.

Many low vision patients can be helped by increasing the size of the print that they want to read or the size of the object that they want to use. The size of a print can be increased by increasing the print size. This increase helps to increase the angular subtense of the target at the eye's entrance pupil, thereby increasing the size of the angular subtense at the retina and the size of image formed on the retina. As the retinal image size increases, the resolution of the object is increased. This type of magnification is called relative size magnification and the magnification provided is a ratio of the new size to the old size. It is also a ratio of the angle formed at the entrance pupil by the original object to the angle formed at the eye's entrance pupil by the new object. Relative size magnification is thus $(M_s) = \theta'/\theta$ or ratios subtended at the retina by their corresponding images.

Relative size magnification = New size of the print or object of regard

 Old size of the print or object of regard

Due to poor vision, many patients may not be able to read the print of a book or magazine placed at a particular distance. If the print of the book or magazine is enlarged by any method such as enlarged photocopy or enlarged print version of the book or magazine, to the size that enhances his or her retinal resolution, the patient will be able to read it at the same distance. Similarly, using the computer and a printer, the magnification of a print can also be increased by increasing its font size to that which the patient can read. See figure 5.1 below.

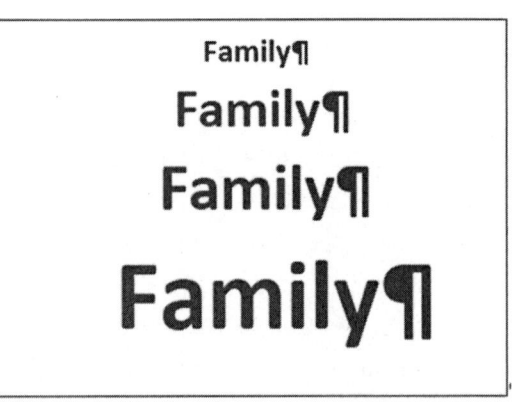

Figure 5.1: Showing the computer generated word 'family' in fonts 20, 24, 36 and 48.

In Figure 5.1, a patient who is not able to read the word in font 20 due to reduced visual acuity may be able to read it in larger font sizes such as 36 or 48.

Similarly, a patient may not be able to see pictures on a 24cm television screen, but if the pictures are presented on a 74cm screen, he may be able to see the pictures. Also, a patient, who wishes to sew with a needle, may not be able to thread the needle if the size of the needle is too small for him or her, however, provision of a larger size needle, may enable him do the threading and sewing.

There are several objects used in activities of daily living, which could be useful to the low vision patient if the sizes are enlarged. Therefore, relative size magnification will enable a patient to engage in vocational, avocational, as well as activities of daily living. Examples of relative size magnification include the following:

Enlargement of print size by the methods such as:

Large print books and magazines

Large playing cards

Large print pictures

Enlargement of objects for example,

Larger television sets

Larger needles

Large size playing cards

.

Angular subtense of the original and new objects at the eye's entrance pupil and their images with the retina are also important (Figure 52). Suppose a patient could not see an object subtending an angle of 30 degrees from the eye, and upon subsequently increasing the angle to 60 degrees by increasing the object size and the patient could see it, the magnification provided is tan 60/ tan 30 = 1.73/0.577 = 3x.

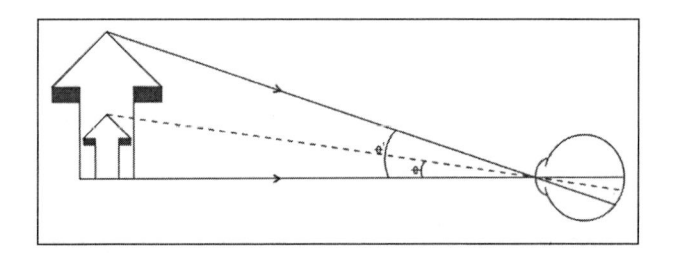

Figure 5.2: An illustration of relative size magnification (RSM), showing how the increase in size of an object leads to an increase in the angular subtense at the eye's entrance pupil and hence in magnification.

If the angles are small, then θ is approximately equal to tan θ and θ' is approximately equal to tan θ'. Also, if the initial object has a height h, and the enlarged object has height h', tan θ is directly proportional to the height h of the initial object while θ' is directly proportional to height h' of the enlarged object.

Therefore, M_s = tan θ' / tan θ = h'/d ÷ h/d = h'/h.

Example: In the example above, if the initial size of the object is four millimeters and the size of the enlarged one is 12 millimeters. The magnification provided in 12/3 = 3x.

The relative size magnification can, therefore, be calculated from the ratios of the angles θ' to θ or the heights of the initial to enlarged object.

An Explanation for the Principle of Magnification

An example of how a patient with poor vision due to central scotoma could not resolve small size letters is illustrated in Figure 6.3 below. Following magnification of the word as shown in the top part of the figure, he or she will be able to resolve it.

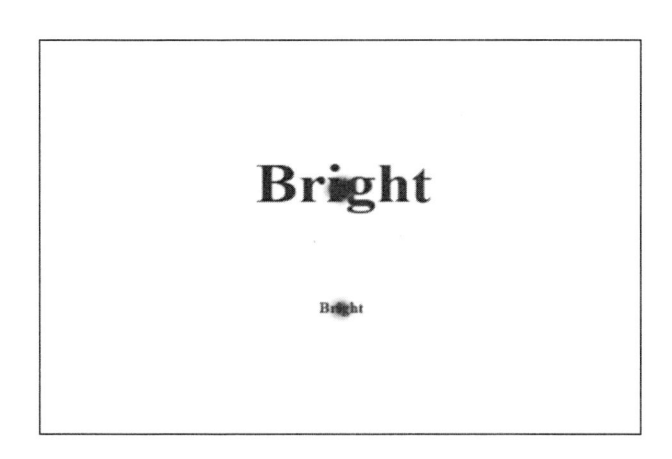

Figure 5.3: Showing how relative size magnification may enhance visual resolution in case of central field loss. In the figure, a magnification of 4x makes the difference.

Relative Distance (Approach) Magnification (RDM)

The magnification obtained by decreasing the distance between the object and the eye is known as relative distance magnification (RDM). An aeroplane or a bird which is far off in the sky, looks very small. As it approaches the observer, however, the size progressively increases. This progressive increase in size is due to the progressive reduction in distance between the observer and the aeroplane or the bird, and a corresponding increase in the magnitude of the angle that the aeroplane or the bird makes with the entrance pupil of the observer's eye. This subsequently leads to an increase in the size of the angle that the retinal image makes with the eye's exit pupil. It is therefore, possible to magnify an object without actually increasing the physical size, by moving closer to the object or moving the object closer to the eye, thereby increasing the retinal image size and improving visual resolution.

Relative distance magnification is the simplest and cheapest form of magnification as it only requires decreasing the distance between observer and the objects. At near, provided there is an efficient accommodative system, as an object can be brought closer to the eye, the object appears larger in size, until the near point of resolution is reached. Bringing the object close to the eye, however, requires extra accommodation or reading add. The possibility of employing this type of magnification depends on the magnitude of accommodation required, the working distance and the subject's amplitude of accommodation.

If the distance between the object and the eye is reduced by half, the size of the object as perceived by the eye is doubled. Similarly, if the distance between the object of regard and the eye is reduced to a third of the original distance, the magnification/size of the object is tripled. These facts indicate that the magnification provided by reducing the distance is inversely proportional to the decrease in the distance between the object and the eye, while the ratio of the original distance to the new (reduced) distance is a measure of the relative distance magnification as illustrated in **Figure 6.4** below.

As with relative size magnification (M_s), relative distance magnification (M_d) can be represented by the equation $M_d = \tan \theta' / \tan \theta = d/d^1$ where d and d^1 are the initial and reduced distances respectively as shown in **Figure 6.4** below.

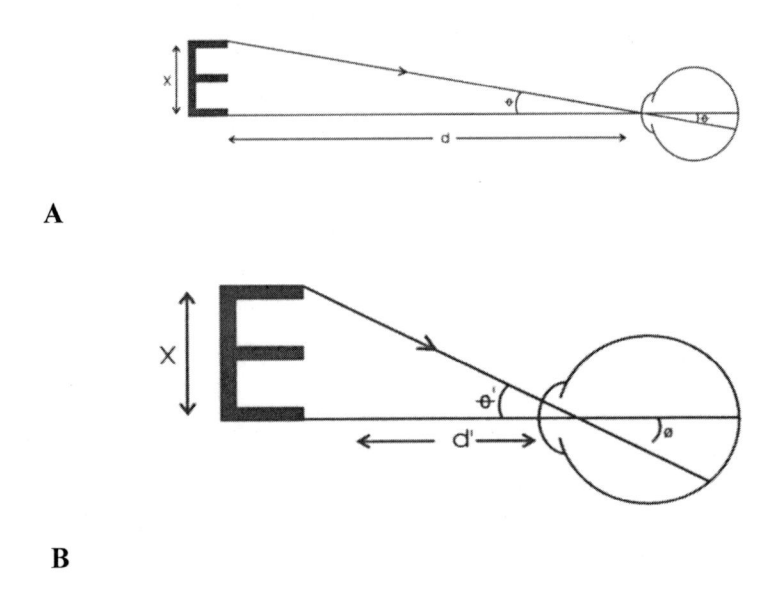

A

B

Figure 5.4 A and **5.4 B:** Showing an object located at a distance d **(Figure 5.4 A)** from the eye. If the distance between the object and the eye is reduced to d^1 **(Figure 5.4 B)**, the retinal image angular subtense with the eye's exit pupil is increased. This will correspondingly increase the size of the retinal image.

A major requirement of reducing the distance between the object and the eye at near is the need for accommodation. A change in viewing distance from 40cm to 10cm would provide 4x magnification, but the accommodation demand would be high and impossible for most adult patients. Many patients do not have enough accommodation for certain distances that they want to resolve printed material due to the high accommodative demand. However, high myopes are at an advantage of being able to meet certain limited demands without glasses because they can work at close distances without excessive accommodation and they should be advised to make use of this advantage. However, many have high amplitude of accommodation, therefore they can move objects closer to the eye, and may not require magnifiers or may require partial magnifying powers for near vision.

The physical reduction of the object-to-eye distance, however, is not the only way of achieving relative distance magnification. The object distance can also be reduced by the use of magnifiers such as spectacle, hand and stand. A high power plus lens such as +10.00 D prescribed for a 45 year-old lady with macular degeneration for instance, may enable her to read prints which she otherwise might not have been able to read due to her ocular condition. In this case, the magnifier used at the focal distance of 10 cm may enable her do her reading. Although such a reading addition is commonly referred to as a magnifying lens, it is actually the short distance and not the lens that is primarily responsible for the increase in size of the retinal image[6,7]. It is important to note that a plus lens will always produce the same size of retinal image, provided the object location is at or just inside the focal point. In which case, the light rays entering the eye are parallel or just slightly divergent.

It is important to note that the use of simple magnifiers at near not only produces relative distance magnifier, by apparently bringing the object closer to the eye, but also provides angular magnification. The total magnification (M_t) afforded by a magnifier used at near, therefore can be somehow represented by a product of the relative distance magnification M_d and angular magnification M_a. Therefore, the total magnification (M_t) provided by a simple magnifiers = $M_d \times M_a$. However, as the magnifier is brought closer to the eye, the angular magnification (M_a) decreases, while the relative distance magnification (M_d) increases proportionally, resulting in no changes in the overall magnification of the system. At the spectacle plane, the relative distance magnification is a more important factor, while the angular magnification is negligible, so that the magnifier acts as a low vision microscope[7]. As the object-to-eye distance increases, the angular magnification increases until it becomes a more important factor. In view of this relationship between the relative distance and angular magnification, the magnification afforded to the patient is constant irrespective of which factor is dominant at any particular time.

Angular Magnification

Angular magnification applies to any magnification provided by an optical device especially a telescope. It is defined as the ratio of the apparent size of the object as seen through an optical device such as a telescope, compared to the actual size of the object (without the optical device). This magnification is commonly restricted to the magnification provided by a telescope. Angular magnification increases resolution through the use of an optical instrument that creates an image; the angular subtense which obviously will be larger than the angular subtense of the actual object[7]. Angular magnification (M_a), may therefore, be defined as the ratio of the angle θ' subtended by the image formed by the magnifier to the angle θ, subtended by the object on the retina without the device[8]. Angular magnification can be represented by the equation: $M_a = \theta'/\theta$, where M_a is that is the angular magnification, θ' is the angular subtense of the image on the retina through the device and θ is the angular subtense of the image of the object on the retina with the naked eye[8].

Suppose the retinal image size of a distant object is x when viewed without the telescope, and the retinal image size when viewed with the telescope is x^1, the angular magnification can be represented by $M_a = x^1/x$. Obviously, this is related to the ratio of the angle formed by rays from the object with eye through the optical device to the angle that the actual object makes with the eye without the device from the same distance. The magnification can then be taken as the ratio of the angle that the exiting rays make with the optic axis of the telescope to the corresponding angle of the incident rays. The magnification can, therefore be represented by angle $M_a = \theta^1/\theta$, where θ^1 is the angle of the exiting rays from the device and θ is the angle of the incident rays into the device[9] (**Figure 6.6**).

The magnification of a telescope system can also be expressed as $M = -Fe/fo$, where M is the magnification, Fe is the dioptric power of the eye lens, and Fo is the dioptric power of the objective lens. In an afocal telescope, parallel rays entering the system, subtending an angle θ, will emerge forming an angle θ^1. The magnification produced by the system can thus be represented by the formula: $M = \tan\theta^1/\tan\theta = h'/f_e = h'/f_o = f_{o'}/f_e$, where M = angular magnification, h' = image height formed by the objective lens (mm), f_e = first focal length of the eye lens (mm), f_o = 2nd focal length of the objective lens (mm). Magnification = $-F_e/F_o$. In a Galilean system, the F_e will be negative while F_o will be positive. Therefore, the net magnification has a positive sign indicating that the image will be erect[9]. Fe = equivalent power (D) of the eye lens, and Fo = equivalent power (D) of the objective lens[9].

Bailey[10], derived F_o and the telescopic lens, for any afocal telescope, where M = 1/1-dFo, where M is the magnification, d is length of the telescope and F_o is dioptric power of the objective lens.

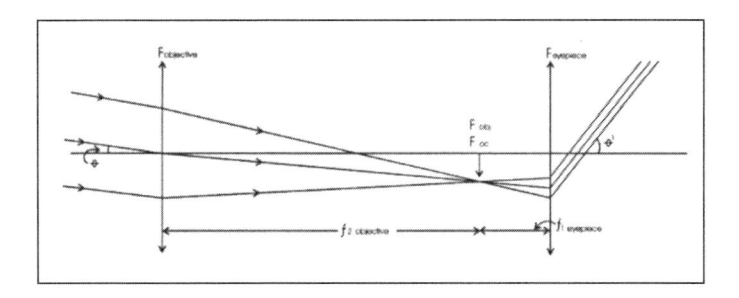

Figure 5.5: An illustration of magnification (angular) in an afocal telescope.

Magnification of Negative Field Expanders

Negative lens visual field expanders are negative lenses of large diameter, which help those with peripheral visual field loss to expand their visual field so that they can navigate easily in a strange environment. A negative lens expander is analogous to a reverse Galilean telescope. The negative lens represents the objective lens of the telescope, and the accommodation or plus Fresnel lens attached to the spectacle of the patient, represents the ocular lens or eye piece.

The magnification provided by the field expander is equal to the ratio of the original field of the patient, to the expanded field is M= tan θ / tan θ´, where θ is the angle of the original field of the patient, and θ´ is the expanded field.

Example

A patient with a visual field of 2 degrees, was provided with a negative lens field expander which increased his visual field to 30 degrees.

The minification provided, M = tan12°/ tan 30°, and is practically = 0.21/ 0.577 = 0.36x.

Magnification of a Telescope with a Cap

When an attempt is made to read at near or view a near object with an afocal telescope, the demand on the accommodation system to focus the image is very high because of the high divergence of rays leaving the ocular lens of the telescope. A positive lens used with an afocal telescope, often called reading cap, can be placed in front of the telescope to compensate for the accommodation demand. The magnification provided by this system, is a product of the magnification provided by the telescope and that provided by the reading cap, and can be expressed as $M_s = M_t \times M_c$, where M is the total magnification provided by the system, M_t is the magnification of the telescope, and M_c is the magnification of the cap.

For example, if a reading cap of power +10.00D is added to a telescope which has a magnification of 2.2x, the resulting magnification M = 2.5 x 2.2 = 5.5x (magnification provided by the cap = F/4)

An advantage of using a telescope with a reading cap, is that the system affords a greater working distance than a microscope of the same magnifying power, but the field of view is narrower than that afforded by such a microscope.

Several telescopes are available which allow adjustment of the distance between the ocular and objective lenses to be varied over a wide range, so that compensation can be made for finite objective distances as well as the observer's ametropia. For the afocal telescope, the beam is collimated when it leaves the ocular lens as well to be focused on the retina of an emmetropic observer[8]. The range for such telescopes can be between infinity and about 20cm. the angles of the incident rays are similar, and those of the exiting rays are also similar. The magnification of the afocal telescope is taken to be the ratio $M = \omega'/\omega$. This is the ratio of the angle that the exiting rays (ω') make with the optical axis of the telescope, to the corresponding angle of the incident rays (ω). The magnification can also be considered to be the ratio of the retinal size when the telescope is used, to that of the naked eye.

The focal telescopes are used at close distances. The incident rays entering these devices are parallel to one another, and make equal angles with the optical axis of the telescope. Also, the exiting rays make equal angles with one another, and the optical axis of the telescope. The incident rays entering a focal telescope, however, are divergent, and make different angles with the optical axis of the telescope due to the short object-to-objective-lens distance. As a consequence of the differences in the pathways of the incident and exiting rays in the focal and afocal telescopes, there is an obvious difference in the magnification.

The most useful definition of a focal telescope, is considered to be same as that for a spectacle lens, that is, the ratio of the retinal image size using the telescope, to the retinal image size without the telescope[8]. This may be represented as M = θ'/θ, where M is magnification, θ' is the retinal image size through the telescope, and θ is the retinal image without the telescope. There may, however, be differences between the actual magnification and nominal magnification of a focal telescope. For practical purposes, the small differences between the actual and nominal differences can be ignored[8].

Projection (Real Image or Transverse) Magnification

This is the magnification produced by an optical or electronic device when an enlarged real image of an object is produced by the device on a screen. Projection magnifiers are quite useful to low vision patients because of the good quality and large size of image that can be produced with them. The possibility of significantly high magnification, large field of view and the comfortable working distance that are possible with them, are their advantages. These systems provide real images on a screen which can be read at normal reading distances. The total magnification produced by a projector system is a product of the projection magnification (M_p) and relative distance magnification (M_d) and can be represented by a formula:

$M_t = M_p \times M_d$
M_t = Total magnification
M_p = Projection magnification
M_d = Relative distance magnification

The magnification produced by a projection magnifier is not dependent on the viewing distance, but the total magnification afforded to the patient is influenced by the viewing distance. This is because the total magnification is the product of projection magnification and that provided by the decreased working distance (relative distance magnification). Because of this, higher magnification is possible without the limitations of visual field and image quality. At near, the use of projection magnifying devices require the supply of appropriate accommodative powers, therefore, the use of a reading additions by presbyopes. The equivalent dioptric power of a projection magnifier can be computed by the following formula: $D = A (x'/x)$, where x' = image size, x = object size and A = accommodative dioptric power (D) contributed by the user. The value A is the reciprocal of the viewing distance, and may be in the form of reading addition (diopters), accommodative power or uncorrected myopia.

References

Bennet AG. Spectacle magnification and loupe magnification. The Optician. 1982; 183: 116-136.

Mehr EB and Freid AN. Low vision care. Chicago, Professional Press, Inc. 1975.

Mazulla D. Magnification for a series of K spherical coaxial refracting surfaces. Amer J Optom Physiol Optcis.1983; 60: 990-994.

Bailey IL. Equivalent viewing power or magnification -Which is fundamental? Optician. 1984; 188: 32-35.

Lovie Kitchin JE, Whittaker SG. Prescribing near magnification for low vision patients. Clin Exp Optom. 1999; 82: 214-222.

Sloan LL. Reading aids for the partially sighted: A systematic classification and procedure for prescribing. Baltimore. The Williams & Wilkins Company. 1977.

Woo GC, Mah-Leung A. The term magnification. Clin Exp Optom. 2001; 84: 113-119.

Long WF and Woo GC. The spectacle magnification of afocal telescopes. Ophthal Physiol Opt. 1986; 6: 101-112.

Jackson J and Silver J. Visual disability. Part 6. Telescopic system 1. The Optician. July 16, 1983; 490-497.

Bailey IL. Magnification equation for afocal telescopes. Optometry monthly, November, 1981

Bibliography

Bailey IL. Magnification for near vision. Optom. Monthly. 1980 71 118-122.

Bailey IL. Magnification equation for afocal telescopes. Optometry monthly, November, 1981.

Cheng AMY. Determining magnification for reading with low vision. Clin Exp Optom. 2002. 85; 229-237.

Dickinson C. Low vision assessment – part two. Optician. 1993; 206: 25-31.

Jali M. The Principles of ophthalmic lenses. 3rd Ed. The Association of Dispensing Opticians. London, 1977.

Woo GC, Mah-Leung A. The term magnification. Clin Exp Optom 2001 84 113-119.

Chapter 6
Prescribing Assistive Devices for Low Vision Patients

The two main categories of devices that are prescribed for low vision patients are **optical** and **non-optical** devices. The optical devices, as the name suggests are those that are made of lenses, and the non-optical ones are those that are not made of lenses. The optical ones generally include those that improve near vision (magnifiers and focal/ focusable telescopes), and those that improve distance vision (afocal telescopes). Magnifiers are only for near vision but telescopes can be fixed-focus near or distance. Also, there are those that can be focused to provide near, intermediate and distance vision (focusable telescopes).

Prescribing Telescopes for Distance Vision

The accurate correction of the refractive error of the patient, is an important step when prescription of low vision devices is being considered for a patient. Many low vision patients have significantly high refractive errors, which if not corrected, will make the low vision device ineffective. Uncorrected hyperopia or myopia will lead to discrepancy in the expected result of a prescribed optical device. Uncorrected hyperopia increases the patient's working distance at the expense of magnification, because some of the telescope's power is used to compensate for ametropia, while uncorrected myopia increases the magnifying effect with the penalty of reduced working distance[1]. As children in particular have significant refractive errors, the correction must be taken care of, before a low vision device is prescribed. Therefore, at this stage of the examination, the best distance correction (sphere, cylinder and axis) would have been determined for the patient as described in chapter 3. Assessment of the magnification required for distance may be done using a distance telescope with the predetermined distance prescription. An appropriate distance vision chart is necessary.

A common telescopic system such as 2.0x, can be used for distance subjective testing. The best subjective corrections (sphere and cylinder) should be inserted in the trial frame, and the telescope inserted in front. This is to be done monocularly, therefore, the eye not being used must be occluded. The better eye must be tested first, and the telescope must be properly aligned (vertically and horizontally) with the visual axis of the patient for effective visual performance.

The need for distance vision device must have been determined, and the preferred illumination level established during the case history. Accurate distance vision correction must have been ascertained during refraction of the patient, and combined with the subjective telescope as discussed above. Also, whether the patient can benefit from binocular devices would have been established after refraction. The power of telescope required by the patient must be decided using appropriate method(s). There are several methods and formulae that can be used to determine the appropriate power of telescope for a specific task. A few are discussed below:

Use of the Best Corrected Visual Acuity of the Patient and Estimated Visual Acuity Needed to Perform the task[2]

The tentative magnification power required by the patient may be predicted using the ratio of the best corrected Snellen visual acuity to the goal visual acuity of the patient by dividing the denominator of the best visual acuity by the denominator of the desired goal visual acuity of the patient. This may then be refined by asking the patient to read a distance acuity letters. The powers can then be refined accordingly to obtain the most appropriate magnification referred by the patient.

In many countries, routes of public bus transport are designated in numbers, therefore a visually impaired person needs to see the bus numbers when travelling, therefore requires telescope for navigation. The power of the telescope needs to be calculated and subjectively refined. For example, a patient wishes to see bus numbers and his or her current best corrected visual acuity is 6/60. If the examiner assumes that the patient will be able to achieve this goal if he or she has acuity of 6/12, the magnification of the telescope that will be necessary for this task is 60 divided by12, which is 5x. Visual acuity of

6/12 is often considered to suffice for most tasks that a patient may wish to perform, hence is often used in calculations. If it is reckoned that the patient can benefit from binocular telescope, that is, if the visual acuity values in both eyes are relatively good and about the same or not more than one line in difference, magnification can be calculated for each eye and the subjective telescopic testing done for monocular and binocular telescope.

LogMAR method[3]

LogMAR or Snellen acuity values can be used to estimate the power of telescope needed by a low vision patient for a particular task. This can be done using the ratio of logMAR steps from the best visual acuity to the goal visual acuity of the patient. This ratio is obtained by dividing the best visual acuity value of the patient by the logMAR constant of 1.2589 until the goal visual acuity the patient is reached[3]. For example, if a patient has best acuity of 6/24 and his goal acuity is estimated to be 6/12. There are 3 ratio steps from 24 to 12 therefore, the magnification needed, is 3x as shown below:

24 divided by 1.2589 = 19.06 (step 1)
19.06 divided by 1.2589 = 15.1 (step 2)
15.10 divided by 1.2589 = 12 (step 3)
Therefore, the magnification required is 3x.
Similarly, Using the logMAR notation, 6/24 acuity is 0.6 logMAR.
From 0.6 to 0.5 is step 1
0.5 to 0.4 is step 2
0.4 to 0.3 is step 3
Magnification required is 3x.

Subjective tests for distance telescopes

It is important to note that calculated magnification values are theoretical values that may need refinement for practical purposes. The next step is to assess the reading performance of the patient with the optical device with the calculated value. This is preferably done with the reading task that the patient wants to perform and with the appropriate level of illumination. If there is a need to modify the calculated powers, this may be done until the best device is obtained for the patient.

Determination of Magnification and Prescribing for Near Vision

There are several methods of calculating magnification power for near, each of which demands that accurate distance and near vision corrections must be achieved first. Practitioners often use distance and near best visual acuity of the patient to predict the magnification power for near reading devices. Final prescription is often based on the subjective refinement of these calculated values.

Kestenbaum's Method[4]

This is based on power (diopters) of addition required to read N8 (1M) acuity. According to this method, the calculated reciprocal of distance VA in diopters (D) will enable the patient to read N8 or 1M print. The reciprocal of the best distance letter acuity is taken as the predicted magnification (in diopter), required to read 1M print at near. For example, if a patient has best distance visual acuity of 6/60, the near addition required is considered to be 60/6 = +10.0D (2.5x). This procedure is not very accurate, but may provide a basis for subjective determination of the power or magnification that a patient would require to read approximately N8 or 1M print. The starting addition for near power can be determined by this method and refined by asking the patient to read a line of acuity letters or continuous text and the power adjusted accordingly to determine the appropriate reading power (D) for the patient.

Best Corrected Visual Acuity and Goal Visual Acuity[3]

The magnitude of near magnification provided for the patient depends on his or her specific need or the estimated visual acuity for the task to be performed. This is similar to the distance method. It is generally assumed that for reading purposes, magnification values which enable the patient to read Snellen acuity 6/12 to 6/15 (20/40 to 20/15) (0.8M to 1.0 M) will suffice for the majority of near tasks that patients may need to perform and are often adopted as goal visual acuity in magnification calculation. Example, If a patient's goal is to read personal letter at near and his best visual acuity is 6/24 equivalent, and his goal VA is estimated to be 6/12, the magnification required is estimated to be 24 divided by 12 = 2x.

An estimate of the print size that the patient wants to read (near goal acuity) and the smallest print that the patient can read at a known distance (cm) will be determined. The ratio of these print sizes is used to determine the magnification required. Example: If the goal of a patient is to read a print estimated to be an equivalent of 2M, but his or her acuity is 8M at 25cm. The magnification required will be 8 divided by 2 = 4x.

Using a Near logMAR Reading Chart[3]

A patient's threshold reading acuity is 6/36 equivalent on a logMAR chart at 25cm, and the practitioner estimates the required goal acuity to be 6/12. It can be calculated that there are four (4) logMAR steps, therefore, the magnification required is 4x. The patient can be given a magnifier or telescope for this purpose or be advised to use approach (relative distance) magnification. If this patient is an adult who has insufficient accommodation to perform this task, a 4x magnifier or telescope may enabled him to read his desired print. However, If the patient is a young person who has good accommodation, reducing the viewing distance by four (4) steps will enable the patient to read 6/12 print. The viewing distance must be appropriately changed using the same ratio of 1.2589 (approximately 1.26) (from 25cm to 10 cm).

Relative Distance Method (logMAR)[3]

Reducing reading distance can produce magnification (relative distance magnification. Provided that appropriate level of accommodation is available, two ration reduction in working distance will produce is corresponding increase in visual acuity performance. Provided the print is seen in focus, changing the viewing distance by a certain factor, produces proportionate change in the print size that can just be **read**[3]. For instance if a child is able to read 0.6 logMAR at 40cm, a two-step decrease in reading distance from 40 cm to 25 cm, using a logMAR near chart, the child will be able to read 0.4 logMAR acuity.

Refinement of Calculated Near Values

With appropriate working distance and desired level of illumination, a device with calculated power/s should be provided for the patient to read the goal visual acuity letters. If there is a need for power changes, it should be done. If acuity reserve is required, it can be obtained by fixed acuity reserve of 0.3 log unit or can be determined by testing for optimum acuity reserve with the patient. There are no significant differences in reading rates and near visual acuity measured with low vision devices by either the fixed or individual acuity reserve methods[5].

Testing for Near Telescopic Needs
Telescopic devices may be considered beneficial for the patient at near, and should therefore, be tested for.

Illumination, Tints and Filters
The best power of device with appropriate level of illumination for the patient should be evaluated, and adjustment in power made if necessary. Tints, filters and photochromic lenses are useful for improving vision in eye conditions such as albinism and achromatopsia where normal level of illumination may result in glare.

Consideration for Prescribing for Low Vision Patients
There are several factors that may influence what and how a practitioner would prescribe devices for low vision patients. Practitioners should be aware of these various factors, a few of which are listed and briefly discussed below.

Visual Disorder Causing the Visual Impairment
What will be prescribed will depend on whether the low vision is a consequence of visual acuity loss, visual field loss or a combination of both. If the visual impairment is caused by macular degeneration or any other macular disorder, magnifiers and telescopes may help the patient, whereas, if retinitis pigmentosa resulting in restricted visual field caused the impairment, magnification cannot help the patient, but may be helped with minifiers, prisms and reverse telescopes, depending on the type of field loss. Albinism cases will benefit from illumination control (decrease) in addition to optical devices, whereas macular degeneration cases will need increased illumination. If poor acuity causing the visual impairment is accompanied by visual field loss, it may be necessary to avoid prescribing too high magnification because magnified prints may be difficult for the patient to read quickly due to reduced visual field.

The Severity of the Visual Disorder
The severity of the disorder will influence the magnitude of the prescription to be prescribed. In general terms, the greater the visual acuity loss, the greater the power of the magnifier required by the patient. Also, the severity of visual field may influence the magnitude of prism that may be needed for field

enhancement. Where a child has insufficient vision to read prints smaller than N24, schools often consider use of CCTV in conjunction with Braille. Braille may be used for speed and ease of literacy, whereas print with the aid of low vision devices will be used for essential information and material that is readily available in Braille[6]

Etiological Consideration

In prescribing optical, non-optical and electronic devices for the patient, consideration should be given to the etiology of the condition leading to low vision. Albinism cases will benefit from illumination control rather than optical device. In view of the macular hypoplasia, magnification may not be as effective in helping certain patients as illumination control. For a patient with keratoconus, astigmatism should be given careful consideration. Etiological consideration is of particular importance in prescribing illumination for the patient.

Magnitude of Magnification to be Prescribed

It may occasionally be necessary not to prescribe the full power determined for the patient. For example, for a new patient, it may be necessary to avoid prescribing too high magnification, because magnified prints are difficult for the patient to read quickly due to reduced visual field. Although a macular degeneration patient may look for really large prints because of the central field problem, with a little gentle coaxing and possibly eccentric viewing, he or she may see small print, and thus require less magnification[7]. A slightly lower power may initially be prescribed for patients, while higher magnification may be prescribed later, if considered necessary. It is best to start with what the patient has to read to maintain independence, rather than what he or she needs to read for leisure, education or employment[8]. It is, therefore, more successful to concentrate on spot/survival reading, even when the patient is able to regain fluency.

Patient's Needs (Task Requirement)

As the patient often has more than task to perform, more than one visual need is required. The various needs of the patient must thus be identified, and appropriate devices prescribed. The distance and near needs of the patient should be taken care of as well. Even at far or near, a patient may need different magnifications for different tasks. A patient who needs a certain magnification to read N8 in a newspaper, may need different magnification to read drug label. Intermediate vision should be taken into consideration too. It is important, however, to note that the need should be limited, otherwise, success may be compromised. A patient whose hobby is playing piano will obviously need a different power from that needed for reading. In addition, the cosmesis of the device as viewed by the patient should be taken into consideration as well. There is no need to prescribe an optical device if the patient will not use it because of poor cosmesis.

Type of Patient

When dealing with a new patient, it may be necessary not to prescribe the full power determined, especially if the magnification is high. For example, for a new patient high power telescope may present difficulty in focusing. It may be necessary to prescribed less than optimum power initially.

Task/s to be Performed by the Patient

Obviously, the type of task to be performed (for example, reading or navigation) will dictate whether the device will be a magnifier or near telescope or a distance telescope. If the patient has more than one task to perform, more than one device will be required. The various needs of the patient must thus be identified and appropriate devices prescribed.

Need for Acuity Reserve

Whittaker and Lovie-Kitchin[9] defined acuity reserve as ratio of the print size of the reading material to the subject's visual acuity threshold for the particular print being read. The higher the acuity ratio, the better. For example, for a ratio of 1:1, the patient may be able to read, but slowly. With a greater acuity reserve, the patient may be able to read faster, resulting in greater reading speed. For fluent reading greater acuity reserve is needed. It is essential that the acuity reserve be taken into consideration in prescribing near reading magnifiers for the patient. However, the adverse effects of high powers must be taken into consideration as well in prescribing acuity reserve powers. If a low vision patient uses a magnifier to achieve spot reading, it has to be strong enough to enlarge a print that is too small, up to the threshold size[9].

Contrast Reserve

Several visual diseases not only reduce visual acuity, they also may impair a patient's ability to detect lower contrast objects that are well above acuity threshold[10] Contrast reserve is defined as the ratio of print contrast relative to contrast threshold of the patient, the print threshold being higher than the patient's threshold[10]. According to Mohammed and Dickinson[11], for the reading task, contrast reserve is defined as the ratio of the letter contrast of the printed letters, to the reader's contrast threshold. Contrast threshold can be defined as the minimum contrast of a print or an object that can be resolved by a patient. In simple terms, contrast reserve can be defined as the extra contrast provided for the patient above what he or she will need to identify a word or read a line. Acuity reserve is important as good contrast reserve enhances fluent reading[12]. So, for fluency in reading, the contrast reserve will need to be high. For instance, if the contrast threshold of a patient is 20%, and the goal threshold is 40%, the contrast reserve is 1:2.

Size and Location of the Visual Field

Magnification reduces visual field, therefore, reduced (constricted) visual field would influence the magnitude of power of magnifier to be prescribed. Also, magnitude and location of visual field loss influences the type of prism field enhancement needed for treatment. Many glaucoma patients cannot use as high a magnification as they would need in relation to their visual acuity[8].

Amplitude of Accommodation

The accommodation status of the patient must be weighed against what is to be prescribed. For instance, in prescribing a stand magnifier, it must be established that the patient has enough accommodation needed for the device. Where there is insufficient accommodation, reading additions must be prescribed to be used with the device. Children generally have good accommodation, and therefore, may prefer to read at a close distance rather than using optical devices at near. Therefore approach (relative distance) magnification may be employed rather than prescribing magnification for children who have enough accommodation for reading. Children with poor accommodation status and aphakes will always need reading additions. As a general rule, any device which permits easy access to texts two or three times smaller than the required acuity at near, should be prescribed[6].

Binocularity

Both ocular diseases and binocular anomaly may cause near vision disturbance that may affect the performance on near tasks, especially reading. Binocular high power lenses (magnifiers) may cause visual symptoms if allowance is not made to assist convergence. For high power spectacle magnifiers, 1^Δ to 2^Δ base-in prisms are usually incorporated above the corresponding power of the dioptric power of the lens to aid convergence. A +8.00D binocular near reading spectacle, therefore may have a base-in prism of 10^Δ incorporated in each lens.

Working Distance and Working Space Desired by the Patient

The working distance (distance between object plane and spectacle plane) and working space (space between object and front of optical device) should always be given consideration in prescribing devices. For spectacle magnifiers, the working distance is usually the same as the working space because they are worn at the spectacle plane of the patient. Telescopes and loupes, however, generally have shorter working space than working distance because the front part of the objective lens is not at the spectacle plane. The working space needed by the patient must be taken into consideration when prescribing devices

Attitude of the Patient

The attitude of the patient towards a device would influence acceptance and motivation to use the device. Therefore, the attitude of the patient toward the device being considered for prescription should be evaluated. Where a patient seems not to like a device, an alternate device acceptable to him or her should be considered. Selection of patients for ow vision devices should be done with care. Mental and physical agility and motivation are more important than visual acuity. A well-motivated low vision patient is he who wishes to perform certain tasks, and is willing to change habits and learn new techniques in order to do so[13].

Economic Factor

The affordability of a device being considered for a patient should be determined before prescription is given. If there is an indication that the device being considered is not affordable to the patient, a cheaper alternative should be considered.

Age of the Patient and Physical Handicap

The age of the patient must be considered in prescribing aids for the visually impaired. Many of the elderly and young children may not effectively use a device that requires a steady hand and critical focusing. Any device requiring hand manipulation should be prescribed with caution for very old patients and very young children. Children generally, have good accommodation and thus, will require less power of optical device for reading. Although, visual devices requiring keen focusing are not generally recommended for a child, such devices should be prescribed as soon as the child reaches the appropriate age for their use. By contrast, certain devices are readily accepted by children than other. Fr instance, many children like the Dome (bright field) magnifier[14].

Fluctuating Vision

Fluctuating vision may occur in patients with diabetes and where the refraction and visual acuity may vary from time to time. Correction values for refractive errors and vision must stabilize before any low vision device is prescribed. Therefore, more than visit may be necessary.

Prescription of Appropriate Reading Device

It is important that appropriate devices are prescribed for a patient. Devices that are appropriate for the age, physical status and preference of the patient should be prescribed for a patient.

Reading Performance Evaluation

Reading is one of the most common goals of low vision patients, including children. It is therefore, imperative that this task be given priority in low vision care. The reading performance of low vision patients should be evaluated following a decision to prescribe a near visual device. Reading performance in terms of reading rate (words correctly read) reading speed (words read per minute) of the patient should be evaluated and recorded following prescription of device/s. This should be done at the visual acuity level at which the patient is able to achieve a fairly good fluent reading. The best spectacle correction, optical device/s to be recommended for the patient and the preferred illumination level should be used in the performance assessment. According to Bowers et. al.[15], reading acuity, fluency and speed should be evaluated with the appropriate illumination level preferred by the patient. Other levels such as low illumination (5-20 lux), normal room illumination (100 to 300 lux), and at high illumination (2,000 to 5,000 lux) could be tried as well. Using a lamp at about 20 cm or less from the reading material. Fortunately, many children with low vision can achieve near normal reading rates with appropriate magnification, while many of the elderly will benefit from optical devices and good level of illumination[13].

Education, Training and After Care
Education

It is absolutely mandatory that patients (children and adults) for whom low vision devices have been prescribed, are provided with enough in-office education about such devices to familiarize them with the uses and other aspects of the devices. Education should include information on the name/s, and the various parts of each device. Also, what each device is used for, and when, where, and how to use each device, should be communicated to the patient. Further, the patient should be well informed of the advantages, disadvantages and limitations of each device. Issues relating to hazards and safety measures associated with the use of each device, such as mobility problems, should be discussed effectively with the patient. For instance, the fact that telescopes are not meant for constant wear when walking should be emphasized to avoid risk of fall. Further, information about the care, cleaning and maintenance of each device should be provided. For young children and the elderly, these information should be provided to an appropriate member of the family such as the parent/s of the child or the children or a relative of the elderly person who may be responsible for the patient's appropriate use and care of the device/s.

Training on Devices

In addition to the education provided to the patient about the devices and how to use them, it is absolutely necessary that each patient for whom low vision device/s has been prescribed, is provided with an in-office training on the use of the devices. As soon as a device is prescribed, training in the use must be given, so that the patient may make effective use of the device at home. The handling and method of using the device must be carefully explained and demonstrated to the patient. For instance, the patient must be carefully trained in focusing method/s. The appropriate method of using a spectacle magnifier with regard to focal distance must be explained and demonstrated. The use of non-optical device such as typoscope must be carefully explained. The site and duration of the training will depend on such factors as the complexity of the device, level of understanding of the patient, motivation and age of the patient, young adult patient may require shorter period of training than a child or an elderly patient. Further training may have to be provided at home and or in the school for children. It is advised that the dispensing of the device/s may be delayed until it has been established that the patient is well conversant with, is motivated, and skilled enough to use the device/s efficiently and effectively. Inadequate education and or training may result in the patient not using the device/s.

Follow-up Visit

Follow-up visits are essential for low vision patients, and patients should be reviewed regularly, to monitor their progress and check whether they are using the devices regularly and appropriately and whether visual acuity levels are deteriorating or stable. Devices may have to be exchanged or modified, or additional ones supplied, if considered necessary. Patients should be encouraged to make contact with the practitioner, if any problem arises between visits, therefore, contact details of the practitioner should be made available to the patient or an appropriate person.

Success in Low Vision Care

There are several factors which can influence the success of low vision care, and these include age of the patient, type of ocular disease resulting in low vision, duration of the visual impairment, stability of the ocular disorder, level of unaided and aided visual acuity, extent and location of residual visual field, education status of the patient, colour vision status of the patient, flexibility of the patient, self-concept of the patient and psychological status of the patient. These various factors are briefly discussed below:

Age of the Patient

Very young patients (below the age of five years) and very old people (above 80 years) may be poor or difficult candidates for low vision care because some of them may not be able to respond accurately and adequately to questions during assessments. Also, they may not be able to achieve the critical focusing need of certain low vision devices. Further, some of these patients may not have the steady hand required to focus some low vision assistive devices. Furthermore, some of them may not have the enthusiasm and motivation needed to use low vision devices. However, there may be a few within this age group that may be good candidates, especially those elderly with relatively sound health, good mental state and those highly motivated to achieve a purpose.

Highly Progressive and Stable Ocular Condition

Certain ocular diseases make low vision care difficult. These include highly progressive ocular diseases such as retinitis pigmentosa and diabetic retinopathy. They have poor prognosis because of their progressive nature. A controlled diabetic patient may, however, have good prognosis. There is no known treatment for retinitis pigmentosa and vast majority of patients gradually, over a period of many years, lose more and more of their peripheral field until they are left with only a small central island of vision or become totally blind, therefore the prognosis is poor with regards to low vision care. Non-progressive or relatively less progressive conditions such as macular degeneration, macular hole often have good prognosis. Also, slowly progressive conditions may have relatively good prognosis. Ocular condition which has responded well to medical treatment and is stable may be of good, for low vision management. Conditions which are not responding to treatment or unstable may have poor prognosis for low vision care because magnification required may change from time to time. Provision of low vision optical devices should not commence until there is a clear indication that the condition resulting in low vision has stabilized.

Duration of the Visual Problems

Patients who recently lost their vision (within one year) may not be good candidates for low vision care because they may not have come to terms with the permanent nature of their current visual status. Also, some of them may still be looking for a cure and still anticipating that there is possibility of having their vision restored to normal, if a highly qualified ophthalmologist is found or that religious or faith healers may be able to help them in restoring the vision to normal. With these types of expectations, they may not be ready to accept low vision devices. Patients who have lost their vision for a long period of time (over 3 years including congenital cases) may have good prognosis because they might have come to terms with their vision status and may accept low vision devices more readily.

Level of Visual Acuity

Good visual acuity has good prognosis, while very poor visual acuity has poor prognosis. According to Freid and Mehr[2], visual acuity of 6/18 (20/70) to 6/180 (20/600) have good prognosis and 20/1000 or worse are not likely to have good prognosis. There are, however, some individuals in between these groups who may have poor low vision care outcome because of some confounding factors, while others may have good prognoses. This suggests that the better the visual acuity of the patient, the more likely that he or she will benefit from low vision care.

Extent and Location of Residual Visual Field

Visual impairment due to poor visual acuity, but with full or moderately restricted visual field have good prognosis in terms of use of low vision devices. They may be able to use magnifiers without the inherent difficulties that are experienced when there is a restricted visual field. If there is full or significant visual field, difficulties with environmental navigation will be minimal, even in the presence of poor visual acuity. With highly restricted visual field, however, (less than 5 degrees) the prognosis will be poor. The patient is likely to bump into objects or other people when walking around. Assistance with visual field expansion may be difficult to achieve. There may be a need for a cane to assist navigation. Apart from the size of the visual field, the location and integrity of the residual visual field are important. Centrally located residual vision is better than peripherally located residual field of vision of the same size.

Education Status

Educated individuals are likely to benefit more from low vision care than uneducated ones as the major assistance that can be rendered to a low vision patient is in form of provision of devices which allow the patient to read at near. Educated patients will always have a purpose and need for low vision devices. The need, zeal and purpose to read will always encourage the patient to seek and accept low vision devices. Also, educated ones will be easy to examine as he or she can understand and respond to questions and instructions easily than uneducated ones. Therefore, educated patients are more likely to be good candidates for low vision care. Conversely, uneducated person has no need for reading, therefore, no need for reading devices, hence the motivation to accept and use low vision devices will be low.

Colour Vision

Patients with good colour vision have good prognosis compared to those with colour vision deficiency. The reason for this is that, if there is good colour vision, it is an indication that the macular is in good condition, implying that the visual acuity will be fairly good. If there is poor colour vision, it may be an indication that the macular and peri-macular areas have been damaged, in which case, there may be poor visual acuity, hence poor prognosis if there is very poor acuity. Those with congenital colour vision defects, however, have good prognosis, because with poor colour vision, they may have relatively good visual acuity.

Attitude of the Patient

Poor attitudes such as inflexibility of the patient to change to using non-conventional reading devices as well as accepting new ways of doing things will make accepting low vision devices difficult. Readiness to accept assistive devices and to adapt to new ways is an essential quality expected of a low vision patient. Inflexible patients will not be good low vision candidates. He or she will not be comfortable with use of magnifiers or telescopes. Also, a patient who have poor self-concept, who worries about what people are going to say about his or her devices will be poor candidate for low vision care and his or her assessment may be difficult. A patient who is conscious of self-image, may not be a low vision candidate because of poor cosmesis of the many low vision devices and the short distance of their use. A patient who cares about how people will perceive him with the use of low vision aids or a patient who tries to conceal his or her low vision status will not be a good low vision patient. One who does not care about what people would say or how he looks with the assistive devices is more likely to be a good low vision care candidate.

Emotional Status of the Patient

Sound emotional status is necessary for low vision care. It may therefore be necessary for the patient to be psychologically examined, and if necessary be provided with psychotherapy before low vision care commences. A patient who is exhibiting severe emotional reactions such as anger, disbelief *et cetera* in relation to his or her current vision status is not likely to be a good low vision patient, hence the prognosis may not be good. Conversely, a patient who has come to terms with his or her vision loss and exhibits no emotional reaction in this regard may not be a good low vision patient.

References

Jackson J, Silver J. Visual disability part 7: Telescopic systems for near (2). Ophthalmic Optician. September 24, 1983; 597-605.

Mehr AB and Freid AN. Low vision care. Chicago, The Professional Press, Inc. 1975.

Bailey and Lovie, 1980. Design and use of new near chart. Am J Optom. Physiol Opt. 1980; 57: 378-387.

Kenstenbaum A, Sturman RM. Reading glasses for patients with very poor vision. Arch Ophthalmol. 1956, 56: 451-470.

Labib TA, El Sada MA, Mohammed B, Sabra MM, Aleem MA. Assessment and management of children with visual impairment. Middle East Afr J Ophthalmol 2009; 16: 64-68.

6. Rumney N. Contrast thresholds in low vision care. Optician 1995 210 24-27.

7. Bower J. Practical guide to low vision assessment and dispensing. Optometry today. Feb. 9, 2001, 34-36.

Nilsson UL. Visual rehabilitation of patients with advanced stages of glaucoma, myopia or retinitis pigmentosa. Doc. Ophthalmol. 1998 70 363-383.

9. Whittaker SG, *Lovie-Kitchin, J. Visual requirements for reading. Optom Vis Sci. 1993*; 70: 54-65.

10. Whittaker. 1994. The assessment of contrast sentivity and contrast reserve for reading. In Kooijman AG et al., (Eds). Low vision – Research and new development in rehabilitation. IOS Press, Amsterdam, pp 89-92.

11. Mohammed Zand Dickinson CM. The inter-relationship between magnification, field of view and contrast reserve: the effect on reading performance. Ophthal Physiol Optics. 2000 ;20 (6): 464-472.

12. Cheng AC, Lovie-Kitchin JE, Bower AR. Determining magnification for reading with low vision. Clin Exp Optom. 2002. 85; 229-237.

Rundstrom MM, Eperjesi F. Is there a need for binocular evaluation in low vision? Ophthal Physiol Opt. 1995; 15: 525-528.

Gould E, Stiff B. The assessment of young children with visual disabilities. Optician 1996 212 14-16.

Bowers AR, Meek C, Stewart N. Illumination and reading performance in age-related macular degeneration. Clin. Exp. Optom. 2001; 84 139-147

Bibliography

Bailey IL. Prescribing low vision reading aids, a new approach, Optometric monthly. July, 1981, 7-9.

Bailey IL, Bullimore MA, Breer RB and Mattingly WB. Low vision magnifiers - Their optical parameters and methods of prescribing. Optom Vis Sci. 1994; 71: 689-698.

Brown B, Reading performance in low vision patients: relation to contrast and contrast sensitivity. Am J Optom Physiol Opt. 1981; 8: 218-226.

Cole RG. Predicting the low vision reading add. J Am Optom Assoc. 1993; 64: 19-27.

Fonda G. Binocular reading additions for low vision. Arch Ophthalmol. 1970; 83: 294-299. Fonda G. Management of low vision. New York: Thieme-Stratton, 1981.

Jose RT. Understanding low vision. New York: American foundation for the blind, 1983.

Leat SJ and Woodhouse JM. Reading performance with low vision aids: relationship with contrast sensitivity. Ophthal Physiol Opt. 1993; 13: 9-16.

Lovie-Kitchin JE, Whittaker SG. Prescribing near magnification for low vision patients. *Clin Exp Optom* 1999 **82** 214-224. Rumney N. Contrast threshold in low vision care. Optician, 1995, 201 24-27. Lovie-Kitchin JE, Bevan JD, Bronwyn H. Reading performance in children with low vision. Clin Exp Optom. 2001; 84: 148-154.

Oduntan AO and Briggs ST. An Arabic letter distance VA chart for young children and illiterate adults. Ophthal Physiol Opt. 1999; 19: 431-437.

Chapter 7
Optical Assistive Devices for Low Vision Patients

Difficulty in reading, especially at near, is a major functional consequences of visual impairment, and a large percentage of low vision patients identify reading as their main visual requirement. Many low vision patients would like to read personal letters or be able to improve their academic status if possible. Many varieties of low vision devices are available which can be used to improve visual performance for the visually impaired. The low vision devices which can be used to improve this disability can be optical or non-optical devices. Low vision optical devices can improve vision performance at near and at distance for individuals by increasing or decreasing the size of the retinal image. The most common purpose of optical low vision devices is to increase the size of the retinal image of an object for the patient. There are occasions, however, when the purpose is to minify the size of the retinal image, such as in individuals with limited visual field, as in those with advanced retinitis pigmentosa.

Optical devices which can be used to improve vision and visual acuity in the partially-sighted individuals include simple devices, magnifiers and contact lenses, or complex ones such as telescopes or electronic devices. For most partially sighted patients, a simple device is what is required. Studies have shown that patients have greater success with simple devices such as spectacles, low-power hand-held magnifiers, and stand magnifiers[1,2]. For distance vision, optical devices that can improve vision include conventional spectacles, telescopes and to a limited extent, contact lenses. It is important to note that contact lenses do not magnify objects, however, they can improve vision where possible in certain ways. Generally, optical devices for vision rehabilitation are often task specific, device for one task such as reading mail, may not be useful for watching television or reading the number of a bus or a house. Specifically, there are two main types of optical devices, namely magnifiers, which can improve vision at near only, and telescopes, which can improve vision at near, intermediate and distance.

Magnifiers

Magnifiers are optical devices that may enable low vision patients to read at near. For most partially sighted patients, a simple device is what is required for reading. Patients have great success with simple devices such as spectacle, low power hand magnifiers and stand magnifiers. Spectacle magnifiers (near single vision or bifocals) and hand magnifiers are the most commonly prescribed optical devices for reading. It is important for the low vision care practitioner to have a good knowledge of the use, advantages and disadvantages of each type of magnifiers that are commercially available so that they can be prescribed appropriately for the patients who need them. There are various types of magnifiers, depending on factors such as the size, power, design, and presence or absence of illumination source.

Types of Magnifiers

There are several types magnifiers which include the following:

i. Spectacles magnifiers: Conventional spectacle magnifier, microscopes and loupes
ii. Hand magnifiers: Pocket (illuminated or non-illuminated)
iii. Standard (illuminated or non-illuminated)
iv. Hand held/desktop
v. Hand/stand magnifiers.

Some of these may be spherical or aspherical.

Conventional Spectacle Designs

Spectacles magnifiers are simple forms of low vision devices and consist of conventional spectacle magnifiers that are head-borne, mounted on a frame and worn at the spectacle plane for reading at near. Conventional spectacle magnifiers are mostly high power convex lenses. They are generally acceptable to many low vision patients because of better cosmesis and permit the use of both hands to hold the reading material. They may be mounted into a standard frame or into a half eye frame. The half-eyes (Figure 7.1A) have the advantage of reduced weight and enable useful distance vision patients with fairly good vision and insignificant distance refractive error. Full aperture frames with small eye sizes have an advantage of providing greater visual field for the patient[3].

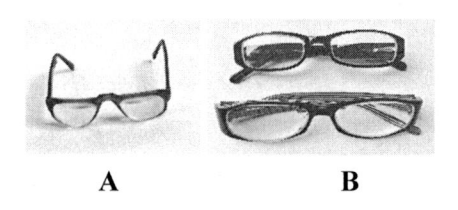

Figure 7.1 Showing a half eye and full spectacle magnifier.

Spectacle magnifiers can be monocular (where there is a need for correction of only one eye) or binocular. Magnifiers can be single vision spectacles for near vision, bifocals or trifocals (correction for near, intermediate and distance vision). They can be prescribed as monocular for high powers.

When both eyes have significant and similar visual acuity, they may be prescribed as binocular with base-in prisms incorporated to aid convergence. Prisms should be incorporated into the lenses of a binocular spectacle to compensate for the additional convergence demands created as a result of high power and reduced working distance. Prism should be incorporated into the lenses of a binocular spectacles to compensate for the additional convergence demand created as a result of reduced working distance[4]. The prism power in each eye should exceed the lens power by 2 diopters. For instance, for a +6.00D lens in each eye, prism power will be 8^Δ (prism diopter) and for a +12 diopter lens, a 14^Δ is necessary. Prism incorporation in binocular magnifiers are not considered practicable for powers beyond +14. 00D. Other options such as anti-reflection coatings may be incorporated in order to minimize reflections for those who are sensitive to light.

Advantages of spectacle magnifiers include the following:

i. Easy to use because they are worn like any other spectacle.
ii. Cosmetically acceptable compared to many other optical devices
iii. Hands are free, therefore allow the use of hands while in use

- iv. They do not require hand manipulation, therefore useful for children and geriatric patients
- v. They are readily available like ordinary spectacles and can be produced by opticians.
- vi. May be prescribed as full or half eye (to reduce weight).
- vii. Disadvantages of the spectacle magnifiers:

- i. Reduced working distance is a major disadvantage because of high plus power.
- ii. Reading material is held close to the eye and this may create fatigue in the arms.
- iii. They have fixed focus and the focus is usually critical for a high plus lens.
- iv. .They restrict the visual field due to high plus power and magnification.
- v. They are not suitable for patients with reduced visual field, because magnification will cause objects to extend to non-seeing areas.
- vi. There may be peripheral aberrations due to paraxial rays.
- vii. Difference in power between both eyes may induce spatial disorientation.
- viii. There may be need for prism to aid convergence for power greater than +6.0D.

Since most children have active accommodation, they are able to read at a closer distance than normal from the eye, and may not require magnifiers or may only require magnifiers with partial powers. Example, if a child needs a +10.0D add (2.5x) an amplitude of accommodation of +12.0D, half of which must be in reserve, the power of magnifier to be prescribed for the child will be 10.0 – 6.0 = +4.0D instead of 10.0D.

Monocular spectacle magnifiers may be prescribed when only one of the eyes is functional or when the visual acuity values differ significantly in the two eyes and fusion is not considered possible. In such cases, they are prescribed for the eye that has the better visual acuity. They, however, may be binocular in design, in which case, the other lens will be plano or frosted. They may be single vision or bifocals.

Loupes

Loupes are generally a variation of magnifiers, intended to be used for magnification at a fixed position relative to the user's eye. They may be monocular or binocular and are similar to the spectacle magnifiers in design and optics. They may be attached to a spectacle carrier (Figures 7.2) or worn on the head (see figure 7.3 for headband). The head-band types have several notching options for head-size adjustment. Advantages include wide field of view and comfortable working distance. The shield can be flapped up when not in use.

Loupes generally provide greater working distance than spectacle magnifiers of the same power and are thus good options when a larger field of view than that provided by a bifocal is needed. The clip-on types are attached to the distance spectacle to provide a full field system at near (Figure 7.2). The flip-up types are more common than other types. When not in use, they can be flipped up thereby allowing the patient to perform distance tasks such as working around.

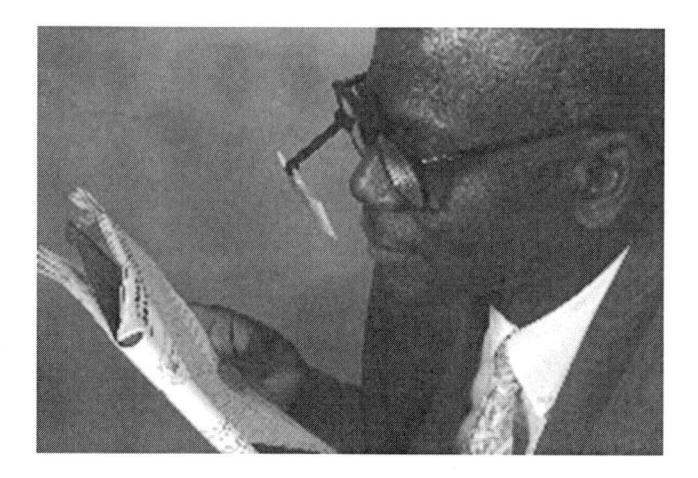

Figure 7.2: Using a flip-up loupe to read at near.

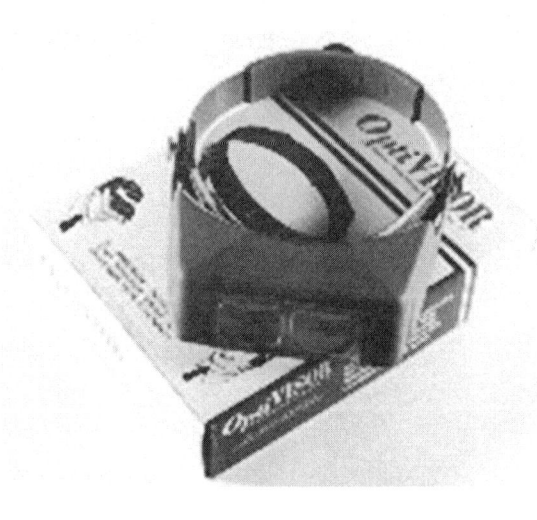

Figure 7.3: Showing a head borne loupe, Optivisor magnifier

Hand-held Magnifiers

Hand magnifiers are hand-held devices which magnify an object at near. They are high plus lenses, usually mounted on a plastic or metal frame so that they can be held comfortably. When an object of regard is located at the focal point of the lens, the imaging rays entering the eye are parallel so that accommodation demand is zero. The magnification provided is both relative distance and angular. The total magnification is, therefore, $M_{rel.\ dist.} \times M_{ang}$. When the lens is placed close to the eye, the magnification is mainly relative distance. This is because angular magnification equation is $M_{ang} = hF + 1$, where h, is the eye-to-lens distance and F, is the power of the lens[5]. When the lens is close to the eye, the h is approximately zero. Therefore, $hF + 1 = 1$. As the eye-to-lens distance increases however, the angular magnification increases. Note that the total magnification afforded by the system is constant in spite of the relative changes in the magnification components. These magnifiers offer working ranges that are greater than those of spectacle magnifiers and are used mainly for short duration near tasks such as reading, writing and drawing and are not comfortable for activities of long duration.

There are several types of hand-held magnifiers (Figures 7.4 A-J). They are one of the most widely used, being the simplest forms of magnifiers and are available in various designs, powers and sizes. They may be in the form of round (Figure 7.4 A, C, E-J) or rectangular magnifiers (Figure 7.4 B and D).

They may be single vision (7.4 A-D, F-J) or a bifocal component may be incorporated in form of a high plus button (see Figure 7.4 E). Also, they could be in the form of foldable pocket magnifiers (Figures 7.4 H-J), in which case, they may have a single lens (Figure 7.4 H, I) or double lenses (Figure 7.4 J).

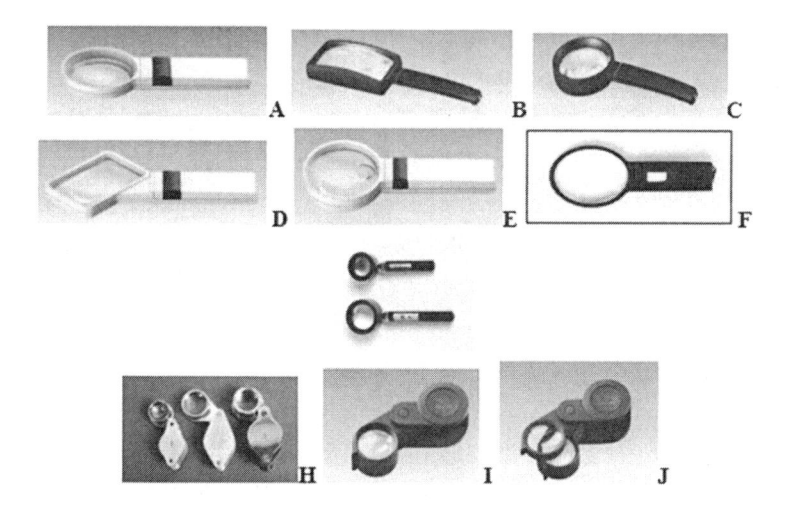

Figures 7.4 A-J: Different types of hand magnifiers

Furthermore, they may be illuminated (**7.4F**) or non-illuminated. Their magnification may range from 1.7 X to 10 X or more. The high-powered ones have restricted visual field, requiring critical focus and a steady hand[6]. Hand magnifiers are made of plastics (acrylic), crown glass or regular glass. Although, the plastic ones have the advantage of a lightweight, they are easily scratched. By contrast, those made of crown glass may not easily scratched, but will be heavy[7].

Generally, hand magnifiers are preferably used with the distance glasses of the patient, although they can be used with reading glasses with a short working distance. In practice, patients often prefer to use them with their near correction in place and to hold the book at a closer working distance[8]. Using hand held magnification with a reading add may decrease the effective power of the magnifier. This is because, the add and magnifier may act as a single lens system. For such a system, the effective power $Fe = F_1 + F_2 - dF_1F_2$, where F_1 = power of magnifier in diopters and F_2, power of add (diopters) and d is the separation distance of the two lenses[9].

If the magnifier is held close to the eye, d is approximately zero, therefore Fe = $F_1 + F_2$, but as d increases, the effective power will decrease. This may eventually decrease the power of the magnifier[9]. Hand magnifiers are mostly used for spot reading such as reading prices on shopping items, instructions on medicine bottles or telephone numbers. With the reading material at the focal length of the lens, the emerging rays have zero vergence. This means that the patient can hold the magnifier at any preferable but reasonable distance from the eye and still enjoy approximately, the same level of magnification while no accommodation is needed. The best distance correction should therefore be worn when using a hand magnifier. However, if the patient chooses to use the hand magnifier with the reading glasses, the hand magnifier must be held closer to the reading material than the focal length of the lens[9]. The effective power of the system depends upon whether it is used with distance or near glasses and the distance where the magnifier is held[9].

The magnification provided depends on the distance between the object and the focal point of the lens. For maximum magnification and working distance, the object of regard must be located within the focal length of the lens. When the object is located at the focal point of the lens, maximum magnification is afforded, the field of view is, however, very small and the depth of focus is low. The magnification provided is approximately zero when the magnifier rests on the material to be seen or read. When the object to lens distance is half the focal length, the magnification is 2x. Apart from the object-to-lens distance, the-eye-to lens distance is also important in dictating the magnification and field of view provided by the hand-held magnifier.

It is important to note that high power folding magnifiers can only be used effectively as eye magnifiers. At any greater eye-to-lens distance, the field afforded will be so small as not to be practicable for use in any task other than identifying a small object such as a number[5].

Hand Magnifiers and Refractive Corrections

It is always necessary to inform the low vision patient whether or not to use the optical device that has been prescribed with or without refractive (near addition or distance) correction. It is no always necessary to use the hand-held magnifier with the refractive correction. It is important, however, to know the effect of using the hand-held magnifier with refractive corrections. One of these is the effect of the combination on the power of the system.

Bailey and Johnston[10] have discussed the resultant effects of the hand-held magnifiers and the spectacle addition or accommodation, and they provided the following formula for the combined effect: $Fe = Fm + Fa - dFmFa$, where Fe is the equivalent power of the system, Fm is the equivalent power of the magnifier; Fa is the power of the addition or accommodation, and d, the magnifier-to-eye distance. The equivalent power of such a system is known as equivalent viewing power, the reciprocal of which is the equivalent viewing distance.

The indicated equivalent power of a magnifier is seldom obtained when the magnifier is used, the reason as stated by Buldoc et al [11] being: if the patient using the magnifier is an emetrope or corrected ametrope, with no accommodation, the patient must place the text being read at the focal length of the magnifier, if the image provided by the magnifier is to be projected at infinity. In this situation, the resulting EVP and the resolution capacity are independent of the magnifier-to-eye distance. However, an apparent magnification can occur, and a patient may report that the magnification is better if the magnifier-to-eye distance is increased. If the patient is an uncorrected ametrope, the resultant EVP will be equal to the equivalent power of the magnifier when the magnifier-to-eye distance is equal to the focal length of the magnifier.

In all other conditions, the resulting EVP will be different from the power of the magnifier. An uncorrected unaccommodating myope, will have a greater EVP than the equivalent power of the magnifier, if he or she chooses a magnifier-to-eye distance shorter than the focal length of the magnifier. In that situation, the field of view will also enhanced. The uncorrected unaccommodating hyperope using a magnifier-to-eye distance longer than focal length of the magnifier, achieves a strong EVP than the equivalent power of the magnifier, but the field of view will be reduced.

For the uncorrected and unaccommodating spherical ametrope, the use of a magnifier-to-eye distance corresponding to the focal length of the magnifier seems to be a good compromise between EVP, field of view and working distance. An important factor to keep in mind is that, when the magnifier-to-eye distance is equal to the focal length of the magnifier, the resulting EVP and field of view are independent of the refractive correction of the patient. So, if a patient chooses this distance, whether or not he uses his refractive correction, has no effect on either the resolving capability or the field of view.

In deciding whether or not to advice the patient to use the refractive correction with the magnifier, it is important to realize that the total power (equivalent power) that is produced by the combination, is not the only issue to be taken into consideration. Other parameters such as the working distance and field of view should be considered as well. This highlights the reason why it is not possible to generalize whether correction should or should not be worn with the magnifier.

Magnification of the hand magnifiers is often based on the theoretical working distance of 25cm, and is calculated in a simple lens system by the formula: M= F/4 or F/4+1 where M is the magnification provided by the lens, and F is the power of the lens in diopters. As manufacturers use different methods of calculation of magnification, different values for different magnifiers with the same magnification specification may be observed. It is important to note that the designation indicated as the magnification of the lens, bears no relationship with the magnification provided by the lens, as the latter varies with the manner of the use of the magnifier[12]. It is never the less important that the reading material is held at the correct distance for maximus magnification. The distance between the magnifier and the object being observed varies with the power of the magnifier. The greater the power of the lens, the closer it must thus be held to the object of regard.

The magnifier is often held at/or in front of the spectacle plane. Moving the eyes closer to the magnifier, will increase the magnification of the material being viewed as the power of the hand-held magnifier varies with the location of the reading material[13]. When the magnifier is resting on the reading, material, the magnification is about zero. When the object is located at the focal point of the lens, however, the magnification of the device is maximized. To obtain the maximum magnification and working distance, therefore, the object to be viewed must be held at the focal length of the lens. For low-power lenses, the field of view can be increased by moving the eyes closer to the lens without sacrificing the maximum magnification of the lens, but this is not the case with a high-power lenses. The greatest effective field of view is present, when the lens is as close to the eye as possible[14]. The patient must look through the centre of the magnifier in order to achieve a sharp focus.

Characteristics of Hand Magnifiers

The greater the power of the lens, the smaller the lens diameter. A low-power lens provide a greater leeway for adjusting the distance between the lens and the object being viewed, but for a high-powered lens, the focus is critical, as there is field restriction. It must thus be used at the spectacle plane. Hand-held magnifiers are usually portable, and are convenient to carry around. They are also less expensive than other magnifiers.

Some magnifiers are made with aspheric (non-spherical) lenses An aspheric lens is corrected for distortion around the edges and are specially designed to reduce peripheral distortions and provide a large field of view. Like the spherical lenses, they are designed for use at a specific distance which must be added to, in order to obtain the optimal clear image of the object of regard. A high quality image is produced when the correct eye-to-lens distance is employed. They have the advantage that, even in cases of high magnification, they allow a greater diameter than spherical lenses; hence provide a wide field of view because of the absence of peripheral distortions.

Advantages of Hand-held Magnifiers:

i. Portable and easy to use
ii. Relatively cheap
iii. Readily available.
iv. Some have additional lens for near.

Disadvantages of Hand Magnifiers

i. Not ideal for very young children or very old adults, as they require a steady hand.
ii. Restrict visual field (this is less so in the aspheric types)
iii. One hand is engaged, therefore, it does not permit the use of both hands.
iv. Focal length is critical, hence high-powered ones are difficult to focus.

Hand /Stand Magnifiers

There are magnifiers which can be used both as hand and stand magnifiers. There are several types of this, including pocket magnifier. Figure 7.5 shows aspheric folding magnifiers (combi-plus) with swing-out handle for use as a hand-held magnifier and folding metal feet for use as stand magnifier.

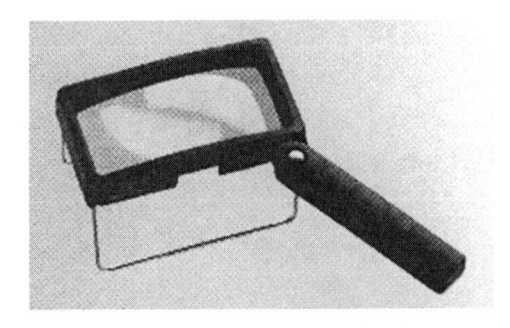

Figure 7.5: Eschenbach folding magnifiers (combi plus)

Stand Magnifier

Stand magnifiers, like the hand magnifiers are plus lenses. They are designed with biconvex lenses or a lens system that is mounted in a fixed position above the object plane. They may be illuminated or non-illuminated. The illuminated ones have an in-built illumination system to provide the extra illumination that may be required. Those with high magnification, have short working distances, therefore, there is a need for extra illumination. They may be designed to permit writing, but are commonly prescribed for reading and other near vision tasks. They afford greater working distance than the equivalent power spectacle magnifiers[15]. There are several types in design as shown in Figure 7.6.

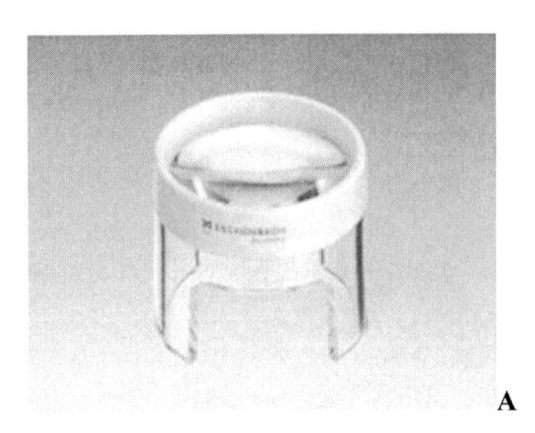

Figure 7.6 A: An Eschenbach stand magnifier

B

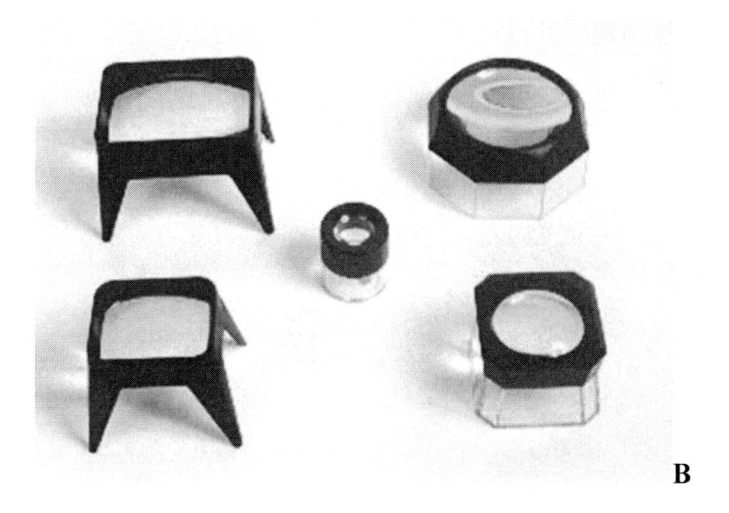

Figure 7.6 B: Different designs and sizes of stand magnifiers

Most stand magnifiers are designed to rest on a page of paper to enable reading. Almost invariably, the lens system of the magnifier is positioned so that the image of the print is not at infinity but at some closer distance. The image will be located at a fixed distance behind the lens[13]. High power fixed focus stand magnifiers should be used in conjunction with reading addition in the absence of accommodation as the stand is almost always less than the focal length of the lens, rendering the emerging rays divergent[13]. The image is, therefore, formed close to the lens and will be larger than the original object so that the image becomes the object. The patient must use a reading addition or accommodation because of the divergent nature of the rays. If the magnifier is brought closer to the eye, the image also moves closer (relative distance magnification) and a greater power of addition will be needed. If the eye is placed at a long distance from the magnifier, there will be a reduction in the equivalent power and magnification[14].

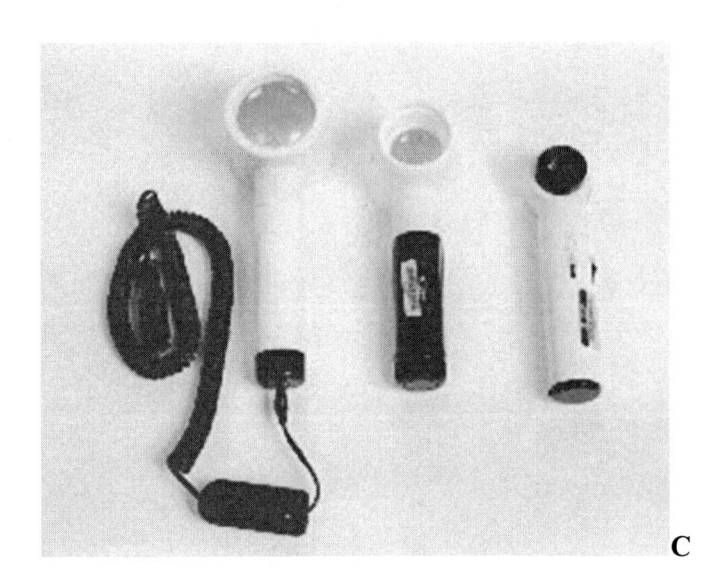

Figures 7.6 C: Illuminated stand magnifiers.

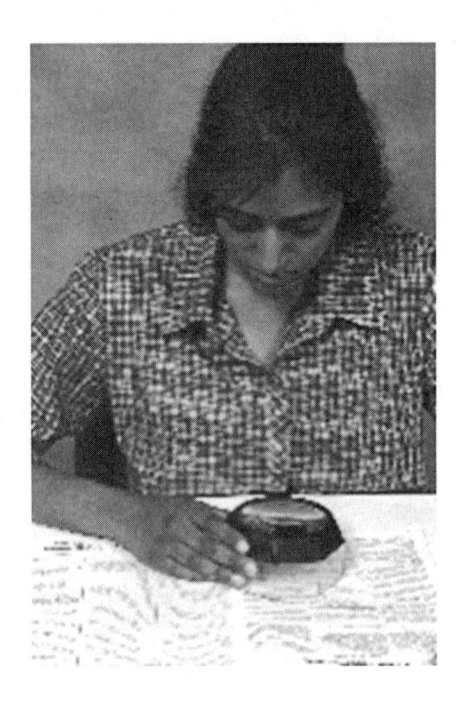

Figure 7.7: The stand magnifier being placed on the material to be read.

Children and pre-presbyopes can of course use accommodation with these magnifiers. Stand magnifiers can be spherical or aspheric, and are generally similar to the hand magnifiers in terms of high plus lenses, but are usually bulky and more expensive. There are illuminated and non-illuminated types. Low powered large aperture stand magnifiers rarely require a lighting system, but medium and high power stand magnifiers often require an illumination system.

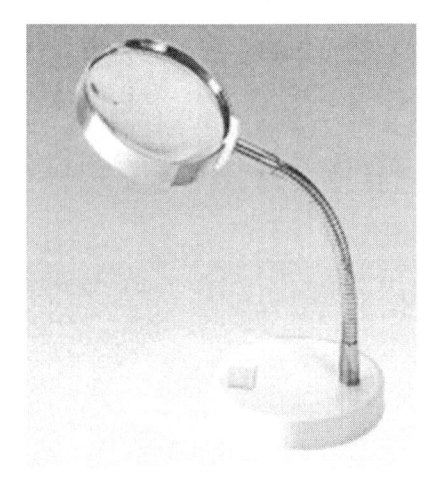

Figure 7. 8: A variable focus stand magnifier.

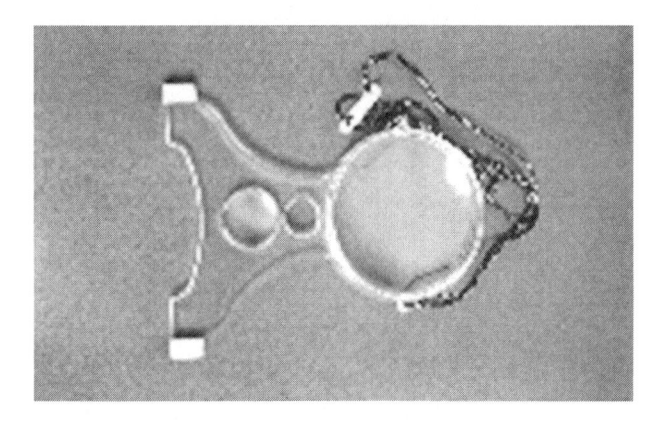

Figure 7.9: Suspended chest magnifier

Suspended Chest (Round the Neck) Magnifier

Suspended chest (round the neck) magnifiers (Figure 7.9), usually 1.7x, are regarded as stand magnifiers. Such a magnifier has an attached cord which allows it to be held around the user's neck. It is quite useful for a patient who needs to do near work requiring both hands free, such as knitting or needle work. The cord supplied with the magnifier makes it possible for adjustment to the height desired by an individual. The material to be seen is held at the focal point of the magnifier. Such magnifiers vary in shape and power, but the magnification is usually low, not more than 2x.

Dome (Bright Field, Paperweight) Magnifier

The dome magnifiers, also known as bright field or paperweight are hemispherical plano-convex lenses designed for use in contact with the working plane. They are designed to maximize their light gathering properties and work best in diffuse illumination[6]. They are available in variable diameters and magnifications.

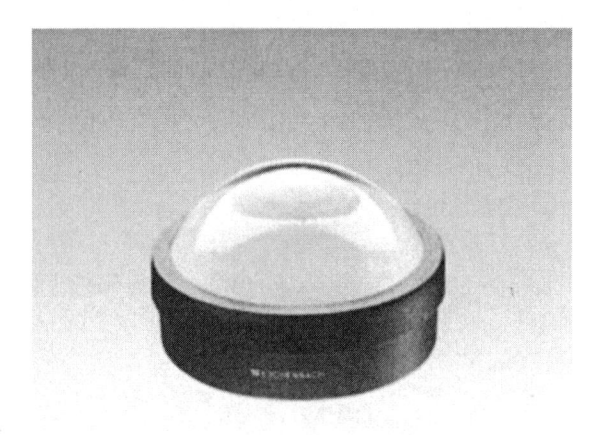

Figure 7.10 An Eschenbach dome (bright field) magnifier.

In addition to round types, other designs are commercially available. The magnification can be increased if the device is held few millimetres above the working plane. They are quite useful to children for reading due to their accommodation capacity. The advantages of the dome magnifiers include the following:

i. Light gathering properties
ii. Minimal aberration
iii. They can be used in conjunction with a spectacle magnifier to increase magnification.
iv. They afford binocular vision and are easy to use

v. They can be used at a normal reading distance
vi. They can be used with a spectacle magnifier.
vii. Useful for patients with a reduced peripheral visual field.
viii. Disadvantages, of dome magnifier
ix. Small field of view
x. There is a demand for a flat surface
xi. Only available in low magnification
There is a need for accommodation or reading addition.

Clear Readers

The Visual Tracking Magnifiers (VTM) or Clear reader (Figure 7.11) is ideal for reading directories, maps and small print. The line reader version (Figure 7.12) is to be placed on the text with the stripe horizontal on the text. The central bright viewing stripe improves contrast. It affords good working distance.

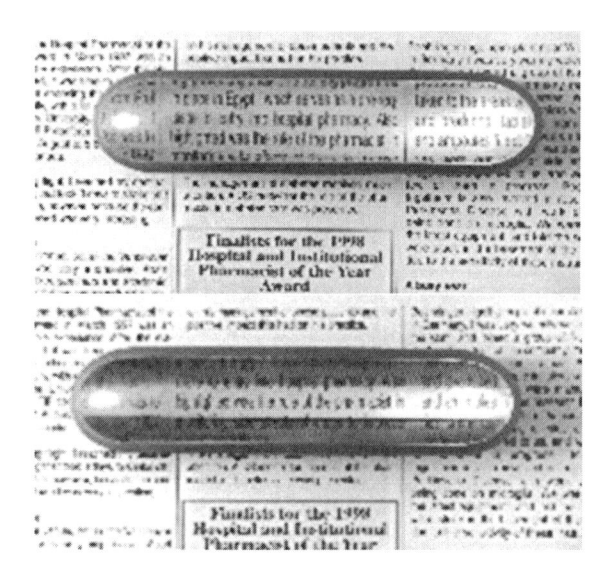

Figure 7.11 A VTM (Clear reader) **Figure 7.11:** A VTM line reader

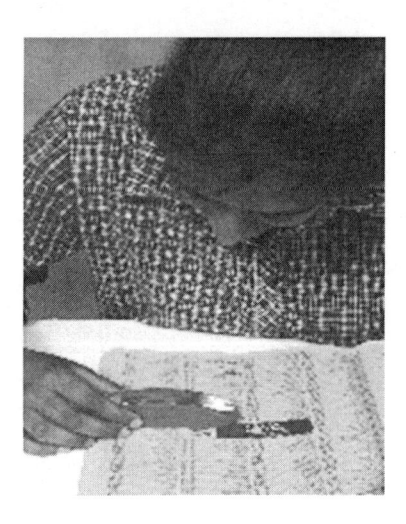

Figure 7.12: Using a VTM line reader magnifier to read a telephone book

Bar (Ruler) Magnifiers

The bar magnifiers are plano-cylindrical plastic moulds designed to be placed on the reading material. There are several designs of bar magnifiers. The bar or ruler magnifiers are cylindrical magnifiers producing about 2x in one plane only. The flat side is placed on the reading material and has magnifying factors of 1.5x to 3.5x. Like the dome magnifier, the magnification factor can be increased by holding it above the working surface. They are useful for long line print.

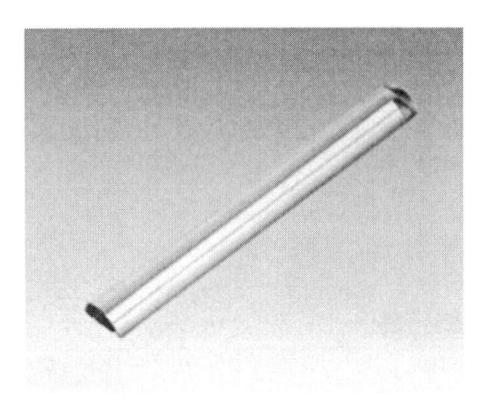

Figure 7. 13: A bar (ruler) magnifier
Advantages of stand magnifiers

i. Relatively low cost

ii. Hands are free to hold the reading material.
iii. They are useful for patients who have unsteady hand.

Greater working distance than the spectacle magnifiers.

i. Disadvantages of stand magnifiers
ii. May be bulky and relatively heavy
iii. They are mostly fixed focus, only a few are focusable.
iv. Patient have to bend over the magnifier in order to use, which may be uncomfortable.

Field limitation with higher magnification,

i. Ideal for short time reading or writing activities only.
ii. With high power and increases in power, the housing height is low due to short length, therefore, the magnifier housing shades and reduce illumination to the text[15].
iii. Bar magnifiers have additional advantages to those of other stand magnifiers.

Advantages of Bar magnifiers

i. Bar magnifier is a plus cylindrical lens and magnifies only in the vertical meridian, thereby allowing the width of print to remain unchanged in size so that spatial disorientation is minimized.
ii. It has fixed focus, hence, when placed on the print, it is automatically in focus. No focusing adjustment required[16].

Zoom Stand Magnifier

A zoom magnifier was designed by Spitberg and Chen[17], consisting of a stationary plus lens and a moveable minus lens mounted on a stand. There are three sets of this magnifier (low, medium and high power). The range of the equivalent viewing powers of the system varies with the power of the add, for a +2.50D add, they range from +6.00 to +23.00D. As the minus lens moves away from the fixed plus lens, the power and magnification of the system increase, but the image remains in focus. The large working space allows both reading and writing [17].

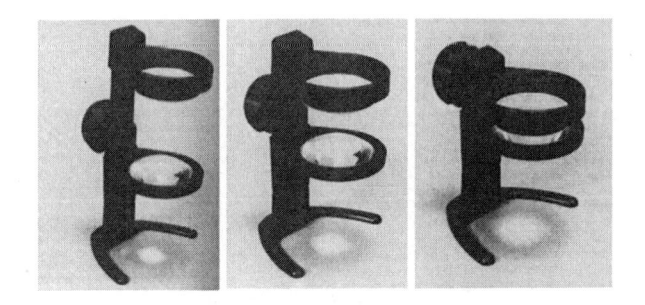

Figure 7.14: Zoom magnifiers.

Advantages of Zoom magnifier[17]:

i. It has two ergonomic advantages over the other stand magnifiers:
ii. It stays in focus (focus) as the power is changed
iii. It has a longer working space to allow both reading and writing.

Disadvantage

i. It is comparatively bulky.
ii. Relatively expensive.
iii. Not easily available.

Reading with Magnifiers

Ability to read is a common need of many low vision patients and for this purpose, magnifiers are the most commonly prescribed low vision devices. It is, therefore important that the magnifier or any other device prescribed for reading satisfies the need of the patient. To read with a hand magnifier, the retinal image of the object has to be large enough and the field of view or reading field width of the magnifier must include enough characters to make reading possible[18]. It is important therefore, to note that magnification of a text in a limited reading field could present difficulties to a patient reading with a magnifier. When the line width and or text height are larger than the reading field of the magnifier used, the magnifier has to be moved horizontally to read the entire text (Figure 7.15). These need to be explained to patients with limited visual fields.

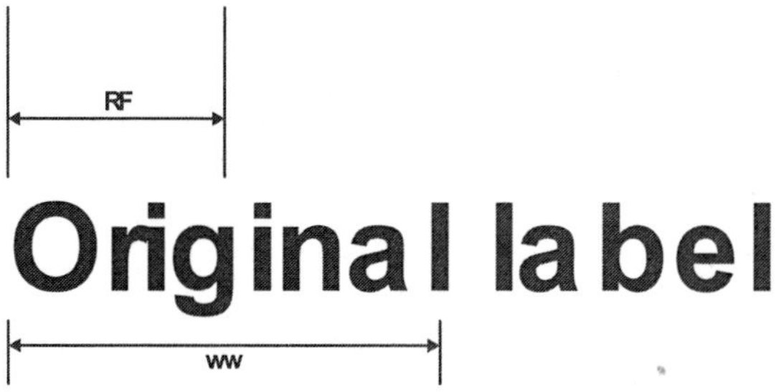

Original label

Figure 7.15: Showing the reading field of a magnifier (RF) and the word width (ww) of the words 'original label' that a patient wishes to read.

Contact Lenses for Low Vision Patients

Various types of contact lenses are available for the management of poor vision, and these include the aphakic lenses, contact lens microscopes, keratoconic lenses, pin-hole lenses and opaque contact lenses. Although the use of contact lenses in low vision care is limited, they are very useful in certain cases such as in cases of high myopia and aphakia and kratoconus. They tend to provide better vision in these cases than possible with conventional glasses. Patient with high myopia resulting in low vision can benefit from contact lenses in that they correct the myopia, enhance peripheral vision and provide some magnification by enlarging the retinal image of the object of regard.

Although contact lenses can be used in the correction of aphakia or high hyperopia, they cannot be used to provide magnification. Generally, spectacle lenses and contact lenses produce magnification in axial myopia and minification in hyperopia. The degree of magnification in myopia and minification in hyperopia is much greater when contact lenses are worn[19]. With contact lenses, the retinal image is smaller than the spectacle in aphakes.

Contact lenses are very useful in cases of keratoconus. It can be used to correct the high myopia and the irregular astigmatism. Compared with spectacles, management of keratoconus can make a significant improvement in patients with keratoconus. Visual acuity improvement from 6/75 to 6/30 is possible. Vision can also be improved in other cases of anterior corneal irregularities, especially with hard contact lenses. Contact lenses are also useful as therapeutic lenses for low vision patients where there is a need.

Individuals with albinism can benefit from contact lenses, because many of them have high refractive errors especially myopia and or astigmatism. Due to foveal hypoplasia however, the improvement in visual acuity is usually limited. Also, due to the lack of pigmentation in the normally pigmented structures of the eye such as the iris, choroid and retinal pigment epithelium, there is light fogging. This reduces the level of possible vision and causes photophobia. Opaque or pupil contact lenses can provide better vision and comfort for individuals with albinism. Although there are reports that contact lenses can cause reduction in the amplitude and rate of nystagmus in individuals with albinism. This may be due to clearer vision provided by the lenses. In their applications as corrective lenses for low vision, contact lenses may be used independently or may be worn with spectacle lenses to form a telescopic optical system. In this case, a high power minus contact lens is fitted for the patient, while a high power plus lens in a spectacle frame serves as the objective lens. This system creates a type of Galilean telescope for the patient. The contact lens telescopes provide good visual field for the patient.

The various uses of contact lenses in low vision care have been summarized by [20] as follows:

i. Eliminate or modify the effects of anterior corneal irregularities or corneal scarring
ii. Providing better visual functions, including visual field than that obtainable with spectacle lenses especially in cases of aphakia, high myopia and high astigmatism.
iii. Produce magnification as the ocular component of a telescopic system.
iv. Opaque or pupil contact lenses can serve as a limiting aperture that will increase visual functions in patients with less pigmented irides and those with iris coloboma.

Contact lenses can be useful for children with low vision. Aphakia resulting from operated congenital cataract is a common cause of low vision in children. The options for aphakia correction for both adult and children include spectacles, intraocular (IOL) and contact lenses. The appropriate option will have to be carefully decided considering the age of the child. Although spectacles are inexpensive, easily changed and generally safe, they may be inappropriate for infants as they are heavy, ugly and create a prismatic effect, visual field constriction, and in monocular aphakes, they are usually impracticable[21]. The options left will, therefore, be intraocular lenses or contact lenses.

The difficulty in obtaining adequate parameters for infants and the subsequent growth of the eye after implantation and the number of complications make IOL less desirable. The life-long nature of the treatment, the uncertainty of the lenses as well as long-term performance are other factors to be taken into consideration[22]. Many practitioners generally prefer contact lenses for infants. While some practitioner may prefer soft lenses for children, others, however, prefer hard lenses. Children will benefit from either soft or gas permeable lenses, depending on which option the practitioner is more comfortable with.

The major disadvantages of the use of contact lenses in low vision care are:

i. Fitting contact lenses, especially for children require more time and effort.
ii. Patients, especially children and elderly, may find it difficult to handle and insert contact lenses because of poor vision.
iii. Compared with spectacles, contact lenses require greater care in terms of cleaning, rinsing and storage.

Telescopes

Only telescopes can be used to magnify distance, intermediate and near objects. The major feature of telescopes is that they can bring a distant object to closer view, so that they appear larger than they would be without the telescope. Telescopes may be monocular or binocular. The binoculars for near may be designed to be adjustable to a certain angle of convergence. There are two basic types of telescopes in terms of design, these are Galilean and Keplerian telescopes. The Galilean type consists of a positive objective lens and a negative ocular lens or eyepiece. The Keplarian has both the objective and eyepiece lenses being positive. In both cases, the powers of the objective lenses are lower than those of the ocular lenses. The Galilean telescope produces a virtual and erect image, while the image produced in the Keplerian is real but inverted, therefore an internal erecting prism need to be incorporated to produce an erect image. Keplerian telescopes generally have greater field of view and longer tube length than the Galilean of comparable power, therefore are commonly prescribed for focusable applications. However, because of the short tube lengths of the Galileans, they are often used as clip-ons.

Most telescopes are designed to increase the size of the retinal image (for magnification). In the case of highly restricted visual field, however, a reversed telescope which minifies the size of the retinal image is used. This allows the image to be accommodated by the residual visual field. In terms of types, other than being for distance and near, telescopes can be monoculars or binoculars, focusable or non-focusable, with or without internal prisms.

Advantages of telescopes

i. One or both hands are free
ii. High magnification possible
iii. Long working distance with near telescopes.

Disadvantages of Telescopes.

i. They are more expensive than most other optical devices.
ii. Bulky and less cosmetically less acceptable by low vision patients.
iii. Focusable ones may present difficulty to children and aged patients.
iv. They generally have restricted visual field.
v. Difficult in terms of training and skill achievement.
vi. Generally, they have reduced depth of focus.

Distance Telescopes

Distance telescopes are those which are designed for used at distance only. They can be binocular or monocular in design. Generally, lower powers are designed as binoculars and higher powers as monoculars, although some binocular Keplerian telescopes have magnification up to 6x. The monocular types are commonly prescribed as hand-held. Also, clip-on types are usually monocular and are designed to be fitted into spectacle frame. Telescopes (monocular or binocular) may be focusable or have fixed-focus. In the focusable telescopes, the eyepiece is usually fixed, while the objective component is variable in position. The distance telescope enables the patient to move around independently by using it to locate desired landmarks, street names and numbers, and bus route numbers. It is also useful in watching television and locating objects in the room. Telescopes cannot be used while walking because of parallax and reduction in visual field.

Monocular Telescopes

Monocular telescopes are prescribed more frequently than the binocular ones. The hand-held ones (Figure 7.16), usually monocular, are portable and particularly useful for short duration tasks. They are used mainly for spotting distant objects and for short-term tasks such as looking at the number of a bus, or of a house or for reading from the chalkboard. They can be used to follow a moving object as well. They can be in the form of clip-on types (Figures 7.17 and 7.18), which can be clipped on to the patient's spectacle frame.

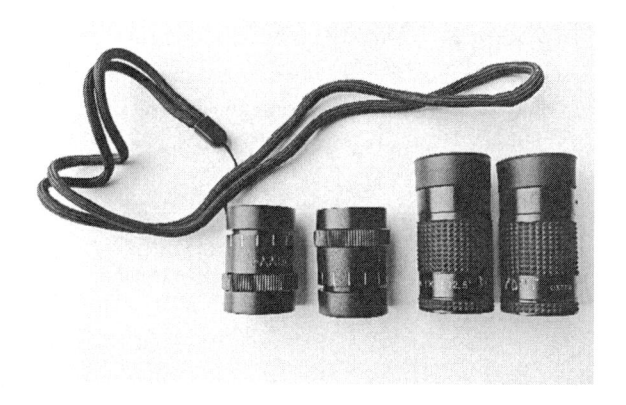

Figure 7.16: Hand-held monocular telescopes

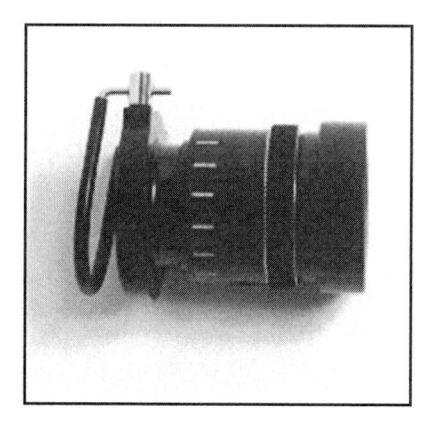

Figure 7.17: A variable focus (focusable) monocular telescope, with clip attachment to be worn over a conventional spectacle.

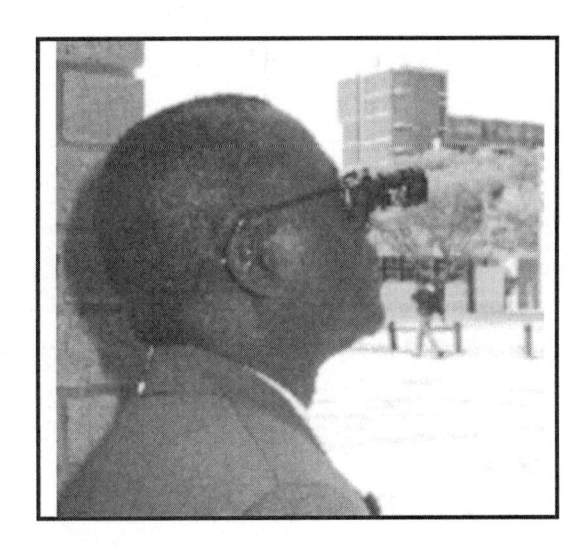

Figure 7.18: A variable focus (focusable) monocular telescope, with clip attachment worn over a conventional distance spectacle.

Advantages of monocular telescopes

i. They are quite portable.
ii. One hand free
iii. Cheaper than the binocular ones.

Disadvantages of monocular telescopes

i. Only one eye can be used at a time.
ii. One hand is usually engaged, therefore, cannot be used for a task requiring the use of two hands simultaneously.
iii. The arm used for holding the telescope may experience fatigue.

Binocular Telescopes
Binocular telescope is prescribed when there is relatively good and nearly equal visual acuity in both eyes. They are worn like a spectacle on the face, hence allowing the patient to perform tasks which require one or both hands. They are however, quite bulky and the cosmesis is poor. They may have fixed or variable focus. Figures 7.19 and 7.20 show distance telescope.

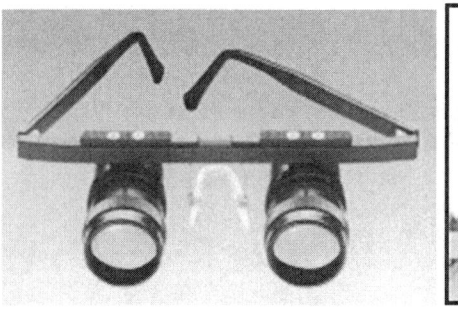

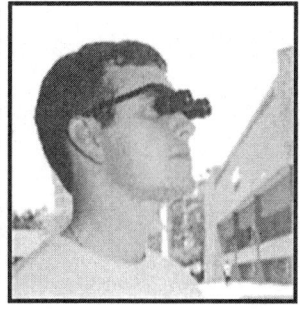

Figure 7.19: A variable focus telescope.
Figure 7.20: variable focus for distance vision.

Auto-focus Telescopes

There are auto focus telescopes, which can change focus automatically as the wearer changes focus. They are available as monocular and binocular systems (Ocutech VES auto focus bioptic telescope). These are head-borne Keplerian types of telescopes mounted on a spectacle frame. Advantages include wide field of view, and continuous focus with changes in visual gaze[23]. They are quite expensive and as they are battery-operated. The batteries need to be changed from time to time, which is additional expenses for the user.

Near Telescopes

Distance focusable telescopes have a range of focus which permits their use at near. There are telescopes that are designed for low vision patients to provide magnification at near and are mostly binoculars (Figure 7.21).

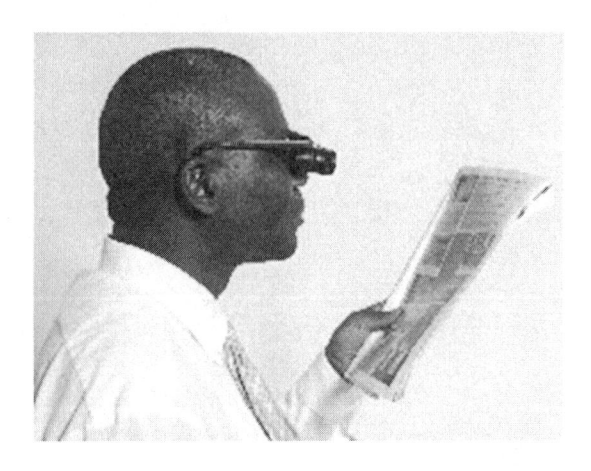

Figure 7.21: Using binocular telescope to read at a relatively comfortable distance.

Near telescopes generally have similar designs as the distance ones, but their optics differ. In the near telescope, the incident parallel rays of light emerge convergent, which is achieved by decreasing the dioptric power of the eyepiece or by increasing the power of the objective lens. They can be Keplerian or Galilean in design.

Tele-microscopes (Telescopic Spectacles)

18. An afocal (distance) telescope can be adapted for use at near. Distance telescopes, usually Galilean can be modified for use at near. One method of modifying an afocal telescope for near vision is to place a lens cap in front of the objective lens. When a distance telescope is adapted for near, by the use of a reading cap, it is often referred to as a tele-microscope. Tele-microscopes are therefore, essentially distance microscopes that are modified for use at near, by the addition of plus power to the eyepiece or by the use of an additional plus lens placed in front of the objective lens by means of a cap. A reading cap is a positive lens which permits focusing at near or intermediate distances. A tele-microscope can be monocular or binocular, and they provide magnification at near at the same time provide a reasonable working distance and working space. They allow tasks to be done at a variable working distance between 20 and 100cm. For more than one focus, more than one cap will be needed which may indicate extra expenses. A tele-microscope may be monocular or binocular. A binocular tele-microscope must be aligned vertically and horizontally so that the visual axes meet at the object to be viewed. The total

magnification produced by the telescope for near work is determined by the product of the magnification of the telescope and that of the reading cap. This can be represented by the equation: $M_{telemic} = M_{tel} \times M_{cap}$, where, $M_{telemic}$ = magnification of the tele-microscope, M_{tel} = magnification of the afocal telescope, and M_{cap} = magnification of the cap. For any telescope used with a cap of +4.00D, the total magnification of the tele-microscope is equal to the magnification of the telescope because the magnification of +4.0D is 1. If the magnification of a telescope is 2x and the power of the cap is +4.00D, the total magnification of the system remains 2x. The focal distance of a tele-microscope is calculated from that of the cap only. Any telescope with a cap of +4.00 will have a focal distance of 25cm. A spectacle magnifier providing similar magnification will have to be used at a closer working distance of 12.5cm. A distance telescope with a magnification of 2.0x used with a cap of +8.00 D will provide a magnification of 4x. The focal distance of this system will be 12.5cm. A spectacle magnifier providing the same magnification will have to be used at 6.25 cm. The advantage of a tele-microscope compared to spectacle magnifier in terms of greater working distance for near task is very important. A major disadvantage is a reduction in field of view.

Advantages of near telescopes

i. They allow greater working distance compared to spectacle magnifiers
ii. They provide comfortable working posture for the patient

Disadvantages of near telescopes

- They are relatively expensive, compared with other optical devices.
- They have small visual fields
- They are bulky and cosmesis is poor

Field of View of Telescopes

The restriction of the field of view is greater in a telescope than in a microscope of equivalent power or magnification. As the distance between the ocular lens and the eye increases in a Keplerian telescope for instance, the field of view increases until a maximum is reached, thereafter, the field of view decreases. Whereas in the case of a Galilean telescope, the field of decreases persistently as the eye-to-lens distance increases. Keating[24] has explained this phenomenon in terms of the exit pupil location in the devices. The exit pupil of a Keplerian telescope is a real image located behind the telescope, it floats outside the telescope. This can be demonstrated by holding the telescope up to a source of light, but away from the eye. A circle of light will be seen. This phenomenon is not seen with the Galilean telescope. The maximum field is obtained when the a person's entrance pupil is at the exit pupil of the telescope. Whereas, for the Galilean type, the exit pupil is inside the telescope, and must be aligned with the entrance pupil of eye. The image of the objective lens formed by the ocular lens is a virtual image, which is located inside the telescope. The closest the observer can get to the virtual image is to touch his or her eye with the ocular lens, at which point, the person's field of view is at a maximum. Therefore, the next option is for the observer to move away from the telescope, and as this is done, the image simply starts to decrease.

Bioptic Telescopes for Driving

In low vision care, bioptics system is commonly associated with devices for driving, usually a distance glasses, and a telescope. Bioptics simply refers to a combination of two optical units in a single carrier so that the units can provide clear vision in two different focal distances for the user. The word bioptics, as the name implies, suggests that the two units to be combined in one system are totally different in their optics. The optics of a pair of distance glasses is obviously different from the optics of a telescope. Commonly, a bioptic system consists of a distance spectacle that carries a telescope for keen vision. When there is a need for devices for two different task positions such as distance and near, or different visual tasks need to be performed at far, a bioptic telescope may have to be used. This may be in the form of a bioptic spectacle in which case, a miniature telescope is mounted in the upper part of the distance correction lens in spectacle the frame, such that the optics of the spectacle and the telescope provide vision at two distances. Depending on the task to be performed with the telescope, the telescope can be mounted on other parts of the lens in the frame.

For distance telescopic use, the telescope is generally mounted at the superior aspect of the lens carrier. The superior location of the telescope allows the spectacle lens to be used for general purpose. Fixing of the telescope is done by drilling a hole into the upper part of the ophthalmic carrier lens and the telescope is mounted there. When the bioptic is designed for near use, the hole is drilled in the lower part of the lens and the telescope mounted there, and used when there is a need for near vision. The near telescopic bioptics are commonly used by professionals such as surgeons. Advantages of bioptic telescopes include freedom of hands for other tasks, and increased working distances when used for near tasks[25].

The telescopic unit may be monocular or binocular, depending on several factors such as equality of patient's visual acuity in both eyes, the need and preference of the patient or the task to be performed. The patient looks through the lower part of the frame to use his or her normal vision for mobility task for instance, he or she then looks though the telescope for magnification needed to view a distant object or print, by elevating his or her eyes.

Before prescribing a bioptic telescope, the advantages, disadvantages and the limitations of the device, as well as the serious training necessary to use the device, must be discussed with the patient. Prescription of a bioptic telescope involves an efficient correction of the distance vision of the patient and a correct calculation of the power (magnification) of the telescopic unit. It is important to note that not all patients who wish to use bioptics will qualify to use them because of the qualifying visual requirements. Like for other optical devices, for effective prescription, certain criteria need to be met by the patient.

Driving, an important means of travelling relies significantly on vision. Therefore to drive, a person must be certified as having good vision. A visually impaired person will not be allowed to drive in most countries of the world. In a few countries, however, visually impaired individuals are given license to drive with bioptic telescope, following a certification that he or she is skilled in driving with the system. Being able to drive around has health implications, and cessation of driving has been associated with health-related quality of life[26]. Following the occurrence of visual impairment, some individuals who have been driving prior to the occurrence of the impairment wish to continue to drive, but can only do that if they can be provided with bioptic telescope.

Visual involvement in driving is a complex process involving visual functions such as visual acuity, visual field, contrast sensitivity, depth perception, ocular mobility *et cetera*. Also, there are other factors such as glare sensitivity, visual attention, visual processing speed and divided attention. However, only visual acuity and visual field are considered for driving licensure in many countries of the world. Visual acuity of (6/9) (20/30) are considered as cut-off standard for driving for the normally sighted individuals.

This chapter focuses on bioptics for driving, therefore, in addition to assisting the patient in achieving his or her goal of driving, the safety aspects of driving are of paramount importance, and are to be taken into consideration. In prescribing bioptics for driving, the criteria that are often considered are the two functions for driving, namely, visual acuity and visual field of the patient. Other important factors such as ocular motility in terms of both horizontal and vertical eye movements of the patient must be taken into consideration. Also, the age, physical condition, driving skill and motivation of the patient are very important for consideration.

Important Factors for the Use of Bioptic Telescopes

The following factors should be considered before prescribing a bioptic telescopic device for a low vision patient for driving: visual acuity, acuity reserve, visual field, ocular motility, age of the patient, disorder that led to low vision.

Distance Visual Acuity

The visual acuity of the patient must be good enough for general purpose, such as moving around in the environment. If the distance acuity of the patient is too low, this will demand greater magnification which may not be possible. The visual acuity in both eyes also dictates whether monocular or binocular device is prescribed. Where there is a significant difference in visual acuity (greater than two lines) between both eyes, a monocular device will have to be prescribed. The distance correction power of the patient should not exceed -10.00 D to + 10.00 D as greater errors will lead to glasses having peripheral distortions.

Acuity Reserve

If the biotic unit is meant for reading at far, it is advisable to give consideration to acuity reserve when prescribing. This means that the acuity to be achieved by the device should be greater than that needed to spot the material. If a patient needs to read material requiring acuity of 6/30 20/100 for instance, the acuity of the device needed may be 6/18 (20/60) to make allowance for acuity reserve.

Visual field

The patient who wants to use a bioptic telescope must have a relatively normal visual field. Bioptics will not be possible for patients with advanced glaucoma or retinitis pigmentosa, as these people have reduced visual field and the bioptic telescopes will further reduce their visual fields. The device is suitable for those with visual disorders such as macular degeneration or albinism (with foveal hypoplasia). Horizontal visual field of 100-120 degrees may be necessary.

Ocular Motility
Although ocular motility is not strictly required for driving, good ocular motility is essential for the use of bioptics. This is because there is a need to change fixation from time to time, with limited head movement. This dictates the need for evaluation of ocular motility of the patient. Both horizontal and vertical eye movements are essential for bioptics.

Age of the Patient
The device is not suitable for elderly patients because it requires critical focusing for effective use, and these category of people may be deficient in dexterity.

Ocular condition
As mentioned above, patients with conditions which reduce visual field are not good candidates for bioptics. Also, patients with active or highly progressive and perhaps unstable disorders, such as diabetes are also not good candidates, because their visions may fluctuate from time to time.

Purpose
Because of the difficulty involved in fitting the device and the stringent procedure in learning to use it, the patient must have a strong reason for opting for a bioptic device. If there is no good reason and strong motivation, the patient may have difficulty coping with the training procedure.

Advantages and Disadvantages of Bioptics
The advantages of bioptics include the following:
They may permit the patient to drive in spite of the poor vision
The disadvantages of bioptics include the following:

- Reduced visual field
- They are difficult to fit
- They are relatively expensive
- They are bulky and of poor cosmesis
- Require extensive training to use

Bioptics for Driving

Many individuals with poor vision will not be granted driving license due to their poor vision. A bioptic telescope may, however, enable such individuals to achieve the desired level of acuity for driving. Bioptic telescopes can, therefore, enable visually impaired patients to qualify for driver's license, hence able to drive. It is important, however, to note that the telescope is meant for occasional tasks such as sighting and reading road signs, while driving and not for viewing while driving. Most of the time of driving, the driver is not using the bioptics but his distance spectacle lenses.

Drivers using bioptic telescopes use their peripheral vision for most of the driving situations, just as do normally sighted drivers, and the telescope is used only to spot signs and to scan distant road conditions for hazards[27]. Drivers who use bioptics use their telescopes less than 15% of the driving periods. When there is a need to resolve fine details, appropriate eye movement is made to look through the telescope for magnified image of the print or object to be seen. The bioptic telescope is, therefore, useful for somebody who wishes to drive in unfamiliar environment, thus needs to read the road signs.

Prescription of Bioptic Telescope

Bioptic telescope is often prescribed for patients who have poor central visual acuity but with normal visual fields and fairly good contrast sensitivity. The telescope is usually prescribed for use in front of one eye only. Significant visual acuity is also desirable. Visual acuity better than 6/60 (20/200) in the better eye, and at least 6/120 (20/400) in the poorer eye without a telescope is desirable and visual acuity of 6/12 (20/40) with the telescope has been recommended, in addition. The use of bioptic telescope should not create a significant loss of visual field[28]. It is anticipated that a patient who wants to use a bioptic telescope should have a visual field of at least 130 degrees in the horizontal meridian. There may also be a need for the patient to have other visual functions such as good colour perception, depth perception and glare recovery.

Bioptic telescopes have been used successfully for a variety of driving tasks, but most effectively for spotting and identifying road signs and traffic signals[29]. The safety concern in the use of the device for driving is still controversial. While some authors[30, 31] reported that drivers who use bioptic telescopes are less likely to be involved in road accidents, others[32,33] are of the opinion, that they are more likely to be involved in road accidents than those not using bioptic telescopes for driving. In spite of these controversies, the use of bioptic telescopes for driving is becoming quite popular.

The fitting of bioptic telescope, especially for driving requires greater care than fitting ordinary telescopes. The training in the use of the device is even more stringent. Apart from the clinical vision assessment, which includes visual acuity, contrast sensitivity and visual field testing, the patient should undergo psychophysical assessments for recognition and peripheral identification.

Training in the Use of Bioptics for Driving

Driving skill assessment should be done using a driving simulator followed by real world driving on the road. Extensive, proper, effective, and efficient training should be given to the person who wants to drive with a bioptic telescope. A major aspect of the training is in emphasising the use of the telescope as a spotting device, with brief but frequent glances into the telescope and spending most of the time in the carrier lens. The patient must learn to locate moving and static objects with the telescope. Tasks to be accomplished during the driving training may include locating stationary objects such as reading addresses and informational signs. Also, training may focus on areas relating to the use of the lens system for driving, such as reading the dashboard displays, maintaining proper vehicle position within driving lanes, selecting appropriate gap distances when entering traffic, locating relevant peripheral traffic control signs, improving visual memory skills, utilising mirrors, and navigating complex traffic situations[34]. It should be emphasized that only practitioners who have received adequate training in the prescription of bioptics, fitting and training should engage in their prescription and training.

References

1.Shuttleworth JN, Dunlop A, Collins JK, James CRH. How effective is an integrated approach to low vision rehabilitation? Two year follow-up results from South Devon. Brit J Ophthalmol 1995; 79: 719-723.

2.Leat SJ, Fryer A, Rumney NJ. Outcome of low vision aid provision: the effectiveness of a low vision clinic. Optom Vis Sci 1994; 71 (3): 199-206.

3.Jackson J & Silver J. Visual disability - Part 4: Spectaccles and head bourne magnifiers. Optician, 1983; March 26, 216-223.

4.Bailey, IL, Centering high addition spectacle lenses. Optometry today, July, 1970: 95-100.

5.Jackson J, Silver J. Visual disability, part 2: Hand magnifiers. Ophthalmic Optician. 1983; 23; 29-35.

6.Bailey IL. Verifying near magnifiers- Part 1. Optometry monthly. 1981; Jan. 42-43.

7.Sacharowitz HS. Options in prescribing near Optical low vision devices. S Afr Optom. 1994; 53:76-84.

8.Logan J. Mc Clure, N. Jackson J. Reviw of low vision aids. Optician 98; 216: 28-34.

9. Sacks, 1992

10.Bailey IL. Combining hand magnifiers with spectacle additions. Optom Monthly, 1980; 81-84.

11. Bolduc M. To use or not to use the refractive correction along with hand held magnifiers. Optom Vis Sci. 1992; 69: 769 -776.

12. Dickinson C. Low vision assessment - Part two. Optician. 1993; 206: 25-31.

13.Bailey IL, Bullimore MA, Breer RB and Mattingly WB. Low vision magnifiers - Their optical parameters and methods of prescribing. Optom Vis Sci. 1994; 71: 689-698.

14. Jackson J and Silver J. Visual disability, Part 3: Hand Magnifiers. Ophthalmic Optician. 1983; 85-97.

15. Goss, GS. Consideration in dispensing low vision devices. J. Vis Imp Blind. 1992; 70: 54-65.

16. Babitz EJ. Advantages of bar magnification. Optom monthly. 1981; 72: 24-25.

17. Spitzberg LA, Chen S. The design of a zoom stand magnifier – A new low vision device. Optom Vis Sci. 1994; 71: 613-618.

18. Neve JJ. On the use of hand magnifiers during reading. Optom Vis Sci. 1989; 66: 440-449.

19. Fonda G. Management of patients with subnormal vision. 2nd ed. St Lois; CV Mosby, 1970.

19. Mandell RB. Contact lens practice. 4th ed. Charles C. Thomas. Illinois, USA. 1988 pp770-784.

20. Levinson, A Ticho, U. The use of contact lenses in children and infants. Am J Optom Arch Am Acad Opt. 1972; 49: (1) : 59-64.

21. Hiles, DA. Intra-ocular implantation in children with monocular cataracts. 1974-983. Ophthalmol. 1984; 91 (10) 1231-237.

22. Green HA, Pekar J, Beadles R, Gottlob LL. The development of the Ocutech VES-Autofocus telescope and a future binocular version. Optom Vis Sci. 2001; 78: 297-303

23. Keating MP. Geometric, Physical and Visual Optics. Boston, Butterworth-Heinemann, 1988.

24. Greer RB. Fitting bioptic telescope: Determining location and mounting angle with bioptic fitting apertures. Visual Imp Res. 2003; 5: 33-40

25. DeCarlo DK, Scilley K, Wells J, Owsley C. Driving habits and health related quality of life in patients with-age- related maculopathy. Optom Vis Sci. 2003; 80 (3): 207-213.

26. Vogel GL. Training the bioptic telescope wearer for driving. J Am Optom Assoc. 1991; 62: 288-293.

27. Bailey IL and Fonda G. Point/Counterpoint. J Visual Imp blind. 1995; 89: 484.

28. Corn AL, Lippmann O & Lewis MC. Licensed drivers with bioptic telescopic spectacles: user profile and perceptions. Review: Rehab Educ for blibness and visual impairment. 1990; 21 (4): 221-230.

29. Korb D. Preparing the visually handicapped person for motor vehicle operation. Am J Optom. 1970; 47: 619-628.
30. Feinbloom, Driving with Bioptic telescopic spectacles (BTS). Am J Optom. 1977; 54: 35-42.
31. Lippmann O, Corn AL and Lewis MC. Bioptic telescopic spectacles and driving performance: A study in Texas. J Vis Impair blind. 1988; 82: 182-187.
32. Janke M. Report on drivers using bioptic telescopes for the California Department of Motor vehicles; California, 1983.
33. Szlyk, JP. Measuring the effectiveness of bioptic telescopes for persons with central vision loss. J Rehab Res & Dev. 2000; 37: 101-111.

Bibliography

Bailey IL. Magnification for near vision. Optom Monthly; 1980; February, 73-76.

Blommaert FJ, Neve JJ. Reading fields of magnifying loupes. J Opt Soc Am Acad. 1987; 4: 1820-1830.

Lovie-Kitchin IL, and Woo GC. Effect of magnification and field of view on reading speed using a CCTV. Ophthal Pysiol opt. 1988; 8: 139-145.

Massof RW and Richman DL. Obstacles encountered in the development of the low vision enhancement system. Optom Vis Sci 1992; 69: 32-41. 13.

Owsley C. McGwin G. Vision and driving. Vision Res. 2010; 50: 2348-2361.

Zabel L, Bouma H, and Mellote HE. Use of the TV magnifier in the Netherlands: A survey. J Vis Impair Blind. 1982; 76: 25-28.

Chapter 8
Non-Optical Assistive Devices for Low Vision Patients

Non-optical assistive low vision devices imply equipment, materials, methods, plans et *cetera*, that can enhance visual performance for low vision patients. Other than optical devices, made of lenses which enable a visually impaired patients to improve his or her visual performance, several non-optical devices are available which are useful for the visually impaired persons. Non-optical devices include those that can improve vision, and those that provide comfort and safety for individuals with low vision. Therefore, any means or method than lenses, that can achieve these purposes for the patient, are non-optical devices. Non-optical devices include a vast array of assistive items ranging from simple thick-nipped pens and thick-lined papers to electronic devices designed for a particular purpose and those that are not designed for such, but can be adapted for the purpose.

Non-optical devices can be classified into visual and non-visual aids. The visual ones can only be used by the low vision patient, whereas, the non-visual ones are useful to both low vision and blind patients. Many low vision patients will require more than one of each of these devices, depending on the type and degree of visual impairment as well as personal needs.

Illumination/glare Control Devices

Visual devices include illumination controls such as visors, side shields, typoscopes, sun glasses, stenopeic slits, pin holes, lamps *et cetera*. A few of these are briefly described below.

Typoscope

A typoscope (Figures 9.1 and 9.2) is a piece of non-reflective black plastic or card board with a rectangular viewing opening which allows the patient to read one or two lines of the print at a time. It is a simple device that reduces glare on reading materials by eliminating extraneous light that may potentially produce reflecting glare on the paper being read. It is, therefore, useful for patients who are very sensitive to reflection from the surface. It is particularly useful to a patient who is very sensitive to glare. Also, it guides the patient on the line, therefore useful to patients who inadvertently jump from one line to another when reading. Further, it enhances contrast on the print being read. The device is simply placed on the reading material with the viewing opening on the specific line being read. It can be made at home for a low vision patient. They are commercially available and cheap, but can be made easily with a non-reflecting black cardboard. The slit size can be made according to the size of print to be read.

Figure 8.1: A typoscope

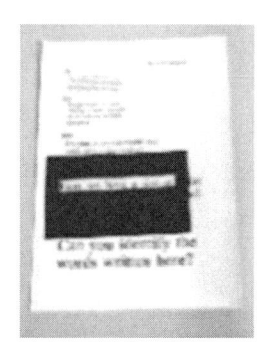

Figure 8.2: A typoscope isolating part of a line on a near reading chart. The surrounding areas of the paper being read are shielded by the typoscope, thereby preventing reflection or glare from the paper.

Visors

These are head wear materials like baseball caps, made of cloth or plastic, which protect the eyes by shading them from the sun or other overhead lights.

They are useful to those who are sensitive to glare from overhead light (**Figure 9.3**). Hats with wide brims are also very useful in eliminating unwanted overhead light.

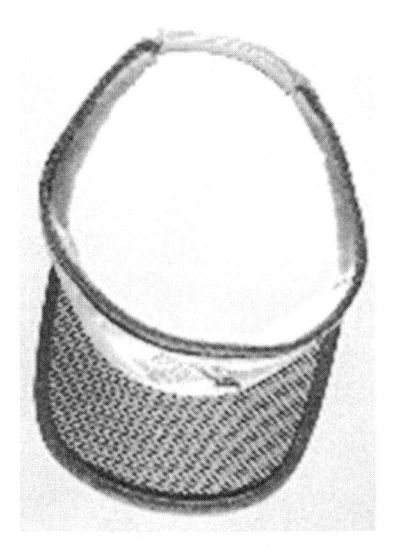

Figure 8.3: A visor.

Sun Shades with Side Shields

These are sun glasses usually made of plastic that have side shield incorporated in them (Figure 8.4). They block unwanted overhead lights and reflections or glare from the peripheral (side) field.

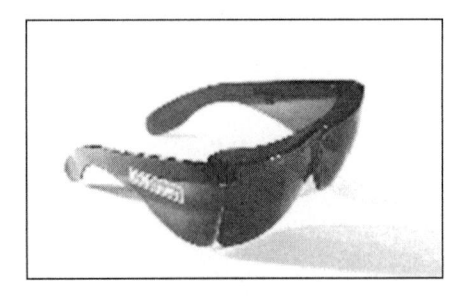

Figure 8.4: A Keeler sunshade with side shields.

Tinted Lenses, Photochromic Lenses and Other Visual Filters

Tinted (permanently coloured) lenses and photochromic (darken on exposure to sunlight) lenses are often prescribed by eye care practitioners to assist low vision patients in maximising the use of their residual vision. This will in turn enhance their performance of daily living activities. Tinted and photochromic lenses will be helpful to low vision patients who are photophobic and or sensitive to glare. They may be useful to patients with macular degeneration, optic atrophy, albinism, retinitis pigmentosa and glaucoma[1]. They may be prescribed in form of spectacle (Figures 8.5) or clip-ons (Figure 8.6). Corning photochromic filters (CPF) in a variety of ranges are available for certain tasks and for certain eye conditions (Reference). People who experience visual problems associated with cataract and macular degeneration can benefit from these devices. Acetate filter papers are A4-sized coloured sheets that are placed over a material being read to reduce glare. There are various colours that the patient can choose from.

Apart from improving visual functions, certain filters also serve protective purposes against radiation damage to the eyes. NoIR™ Sun shades have a range of UV shield and filters that are useful to low vision patients, especially in cases of aphakia. Visual disturbance index (VDI) is reduced by short wavelength light absorbance filters in retinitis pigmentosa patients[2]. Ultraviolet and partly blue-light-blocking filters are used in eyeglasses for patients with aphakia, macular dystrophies, retinitis pigmentosa and other diseases of the retina. There are reports that red glass filters improves visual acuity in people with retinitis pigmentosa. Individuals with albinism may benefit from various shades of filters ranging from dark tints to red.

Where there are indications of reduced light and dark adaptations, tints are preferable to photochromics, because the patient can benefit from the shade as soon as he or she enters the sun from dark environment, vice versa. It takes some time for photochromic lenses to be effective, and the patient can face difficulties when he or she moves into a very bright area.

Filters are useful in improving the quality of vision. They are particularly useful where there is a preference for a certain wavelength of light. It has been suggested that some types of pigmentary retinal degeneration may be exacerbated by prolonged exposure to wavelengths around 400 nm (blue light region. Appropriate filters will, therefore, be valuable. *Retinitis pigmentosa* patients often prefer tinted or photochromic lenses. There are reports that they generally have preference for red photochromic lenses. Short wavelength-absorbing filters are able to reduce light scatter in the ocular media. Thus, they produce an improvement in visual performance in ocular conditions such as iris *coloboma*, cataract, corneal opacity, albinism, macula hypoplasia, macula dystrophies, *retinitis pigmentosa*, and other retinal diseases.

Filters help to reduce light scatter, thereby improving visual functions such as visual acuity and contrast sensitivity. They help to reduce glare thereby providing comfort, and also aid in reducing chromatic aberrations. In aphakia, there is a risk of retinal damage as the retina becomes more accessible to short wavelengths such as the ultraviolet and the blue light. Aphakes will thus benefit from short wavelength filters. Individuals with albinism will in turn benefit from dark amber filters as they reduce light intensity and diminish adverse visual phenomena and difficulties. Yellow and orange filters can improve the quality of the retinal image in case of media opacities because they decrease light scattering in the ocular media. The selection of appropriate filters and tints should be based on the preference of the patient, so that he or she should be tested with various types of tints and filters. The filter should be tested under real conditions, indoors and outdoors.

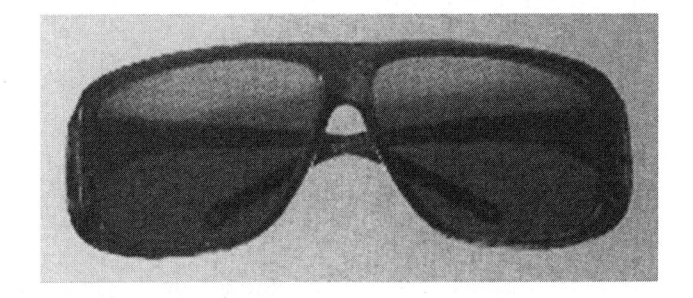

Figure 8.5: Tinted glasses

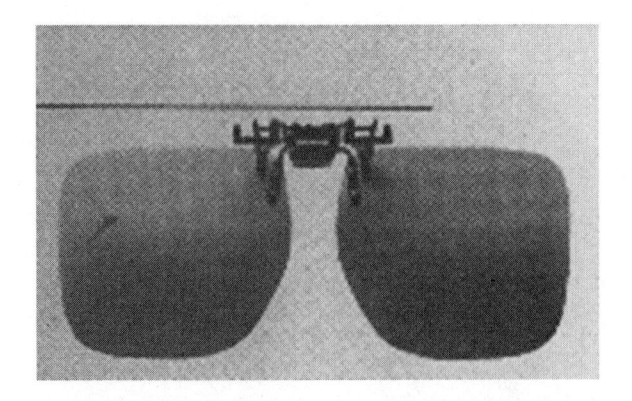

Figure 8.6: Filter clip-ons

Pin holes (Single and multiple) spectacles

These are spectacle shades with single or multiple pinholes (Figure 8.7) Pin holes help to reduce the amount of light entering the eye, and also help to reduce the area of the media partaking in refraction, thereby improving the image quality. A major disadvantage is poor cosmesis.

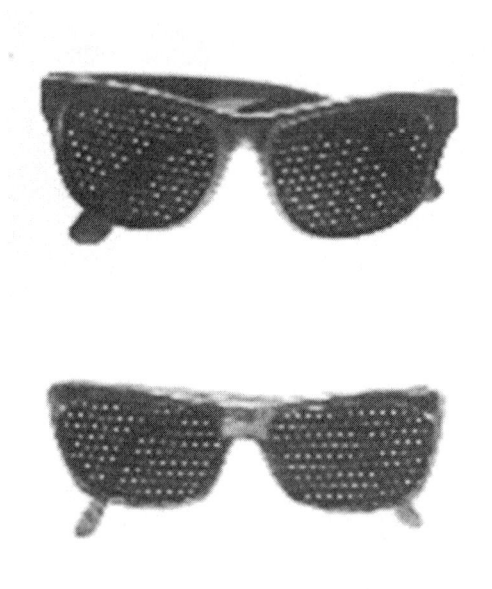

Figure 8.7: Pin hole spectacles

Reading and Writing Devices

Devices for reading and writing include acetate filters, large print materials, reading stand, reading video magnifiers and computer programmes, thick-nipped felt pens, bold and wide-lined papers.

Bold Felt Pens and Bold Lined Papers

These (Figure 8.8) enable a partially sighted person to read and write bold letters or figures. The bold line papers usually have wide spaces to guide the low vision patient to write straight on the paper. The letter-writing guide enables the patient to write along a straight line and afford proper line spacing. They are useful for writing personal mails, and are useful to both children and adults.

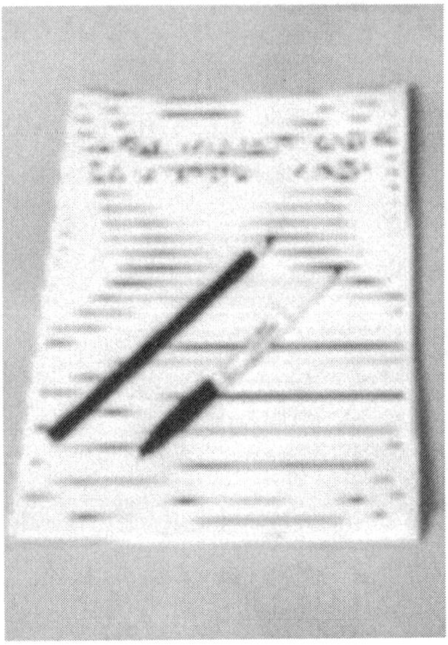

Figure 9.8: Bold-line paper and felt-tipped pens.

Large-print Books, Publications and Newspapers

There are many books printed in large print, so that the low vision patient may not require a magnifier to read them or use a magnifier to increase the magnification when there is a need. These include religious books, fiction and non-fiction books. Photocopiers can be used to increase the sizes of printed material. Computers and printers can be used to generate large print sizes by using large fonts.

Advantages of Large Print Material

The major advantages of the large printed materials include:

- They can be used at a normal reading distance.
- No restricted working distance and visual field.
- Provide comfortable reading distances
- Unrestricted visual field
- They provide good contrast
- Disadvantages of large print material
- The major disadvantages[3] of large print materials such as books include the following:

- They are usually bulky
- They are usually expensive.
- Not readily available.
- Their magnification is usually limited to about 2.0 to 3 times.

Many common large-print textbooks are only found in major libraries or in low vision centres. Some religious books are produced with relatively large prints. Figure 8.9 below shows a large print bible.

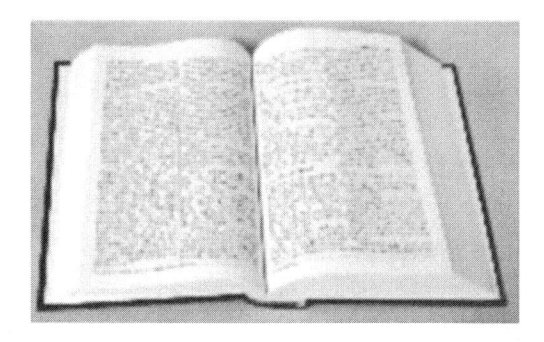

Figure 8.9: A large-print bible that can be read by some partially sighted patients.

Reading Stand

It is often necessary for the low vision patient to hold the reading materials very close and at a particular orientation, especially when using spectacle magnifiers or in certain visual field losses. The low vision patient generally reads slower than the normally sighted. Also, many low vision patients are elderly, and many may not be able to hold reading materials for a long period. Others have unsteady hands; therefore, holding books at a close reading distance can be tiring and uncomfortable. They, therefore, always find reading stands very useful. Reading stands (Figure 8.10) are especially useful when a large size book is being read as this will be uncomfortable to be hand-held for a long time. There are many types of commercially available reading stands. Some are made of wood and others of metals. They can be custom-made.

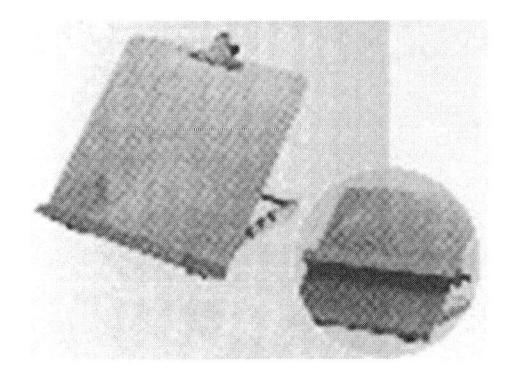

Figure 8.10: Wooden reading stands (Reproduced with permission from Eschenbach)

Devices Needed for Daily Living Activities

Devices needed for activities of daily living include canes, needle threaders, large-format telephone dials, large-print cheques, large-print playing cards; auditory aids such as audio-tapes, talking watches, clocks and calculators. Kitchen aids such as cutting guides, liquid level gauges and walking-assisted canes.

Playing Cards

Large number or digit cards (Figure 8.11) are useful for low vision patients who want to play cards. The partially sighted person can play with other partially sighted persons or normally sighted persons. The bold-print figures on the cards allow the partially sighted person to see the numbers and other prints on the cards.

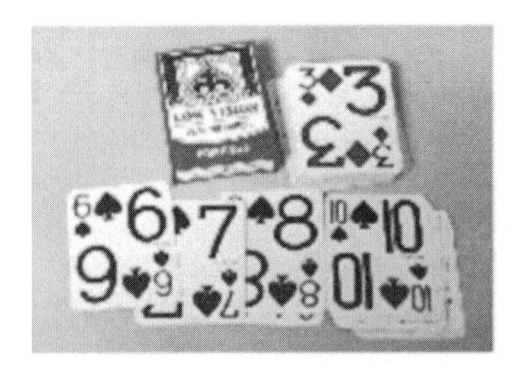

Figure 8.11: Large digit playing cards.

Audio or Taped Material

These are useful to both low vision and blind individuals. Text materials such as lectures can be recorded for the visually impaired and then be played afterwards by him or her. Several books and other resource materials in different languages are available in audio cassettes. Religious organizations frequently use audio cassettes for passing messages to those who cannot or who have difficulty in visually receiving religious messages. Figures 9.12 shows a set of Christian audio tapes titled 'Faith comes by hearing'. There are many types of religious audio tapes. Aurora Ministries Bible Alliance has many Christian audio tapes, which are available in over 50 languages and are supplied to low vision and blind persons free of charge. (Available from: Aurora Ministries Bible Alliance, P. O. Box 621, Bradento, Florida 34206, USA). In institutions of higher education, some lecturers present their lectures in form of audiotapes and distribute them to the visually impaired. Such study materials help the student to augment what he or she heard in the classroom.

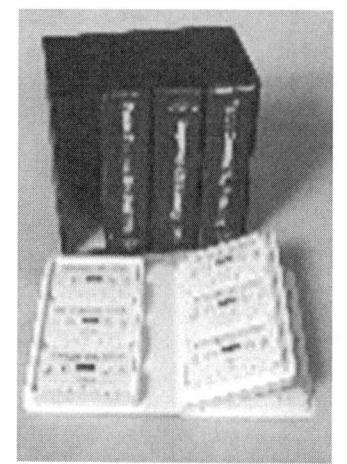

Figure 9.12. A series of Christian audio tapes

Talking watches and clocks

Talking wrist (Figures 8.13) watches are particularly useful to both the low vision patient and the blind. They tell the time at regular intervals and when needed. These are commercially available in many designs.

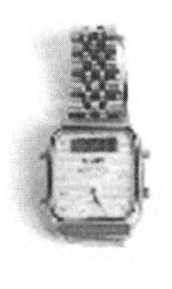

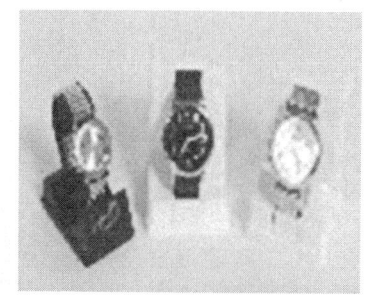

Figure 9.13: A variety of talking wristwatches

Talking Clocks

Talking clocks Figure 8.14, like the talking watches tell time of the day at regular interval or may tell the time when required to do so.

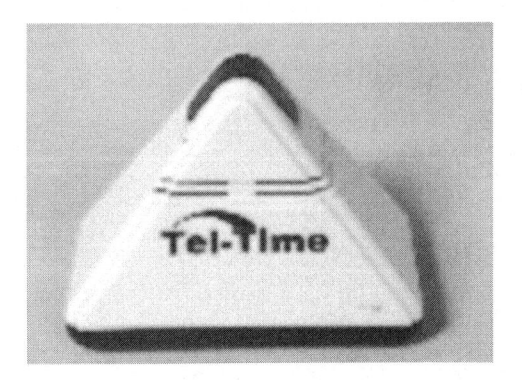

Figure 8.14: A Tel-Time clock.

Talking Calculators

Taking calculator (**Figure 8.15**) is useful to both the partially sighted and blind persons. When each button is pressed, the calculator tells the number or sign that the button represents. Also, when an operation is done with the calculator, it tells the answer of the operation.

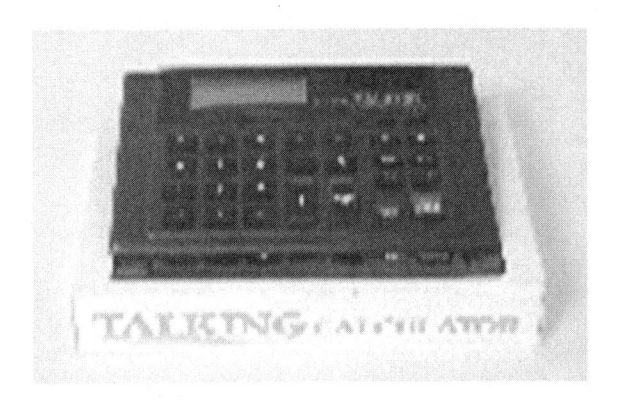

Figure 8.15: A talking calculator

Walking Assistive Canes

Canes are useful to both low vision and blind individuals for navigation. The blind persons use them for navigation, and to detect obstacles on the way. For the low vision patient, the cane may be for occasional use where the illumination available is not high enough for him or her to move around visually or to locate obstacles easily. They are also useful to the low vision patient when there is a need to walk faster, during which they depend on canes. There are various sizes and shapes of canes and are either straight (non-collapsible) or collapsible. The straight ones are preferable to patients who need them always, but the collapsible ones (**Figure 8.16**) can be used by those who need them occasionally. Because of the portability of the collapsible ones however, many individuals prefer them. They are particularly useful to patients who have to travel part of their journey in a car or train, as they can easily be collapsed and kept in a bag or hand-held in the car or train without disturbance to other passengers. Some low vision patients do not like cane as they are seen as symbols of blindness.

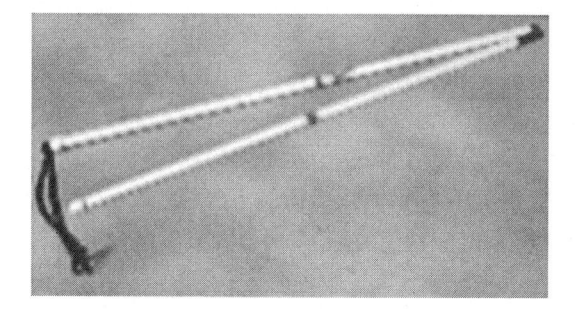

Figure 8.16: A collapsible cane.

Electronic Devices

Several varieties of electronic vision-enhancement devices are available for low vision patients. These include closed circuit television (CCTV), video magnifiers and computer-assistive devices. Electronic devices are a part of reading aids. Many low vision patients can benefit from electronically enlarged prints projected on the screen or from speech output corresponding to the text on the screen. For some low vision patients, especially those with extensive macular degeneration, there may be a stage at which any form of magnification provided by optical devices will not be able to efficiently provide the magnification or the reading duration that they require. In such cases, closed-circuit television (CCTV) or a video magnifier is the only device that can offer the combinations of high magnification, wide-reading field, and enhanced contrast. Reversed polarity (contrast polarity) may also be provided. Reversed or contrast polarity enables black print to be provided on white background or white print on black background as preferred by the patient.

Electronic devices include closed-circuit television systems (CCTV), hand-held cameras, adaptive computer hardware and software, as well as head-mount video devices (HMVD). The facilities provided by some of these devices may include autofocus, relative size magnification, contrast enhancement and reversed polarity functions.

Examples of electronic devices:
Closed circuit television (CCTV): for example Tieman CCTV.
Hand-held cameras: for example Keeler Max video magnifier.
Head-mount system: Low vision enhancement system (LVES)
Computer programme such as zoom text version 70, Jaws version 33.

Closed Circuit Television

The-closed circuit television (CCTV) consists of a camera, zoom lens, TV monitor (screen), mounted stand and a light source. It enables the low vision patient to read enlarged printed or handwritten materials on the screen. In addition to reading or writing, other activities such as threading a needle may be performed on the CCTV. Most of these have in-built cameras which can be moved horizontally in many directions to enable the reader navigate one page of the reading material at a time. The monitor may have anti-glare coating to reduce reflection and increase contrast. Many types of CCTV are commercially available and include portable ones, which can easily be carried from place to place.

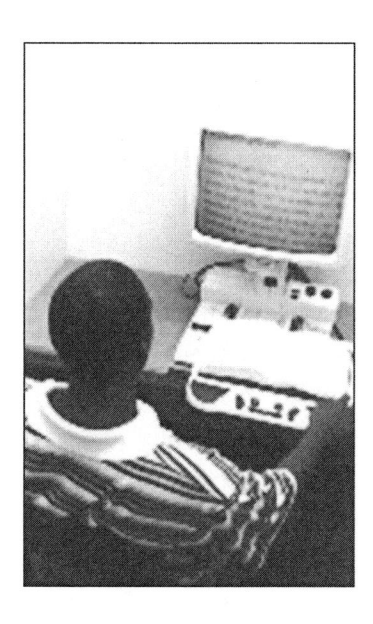

Figure 8.17: A Tieman close circuit televisions (CCTV) being used by a low vision student to read a textbook.

The Tieman CCTV shown above consists of a high resolution monochrome monitor with X/Y sliding table on which the text to be read can be placed.

Advantages and disadvantages of CCTV.

The major advantages of a CCTV include:

Greater contrast enhancement compared with the optical device providing a similar magnification. This is because the various aberrations inherent in the optical devices are absent in the electronic devices such as the CCTV.

They afford contrast or image reversal (black on white or white on black images).

This form of magnification is normally more acceptable in appearance than those provided by optical aids, especially for those using it at school or at the workplace. Binocular viewing is possible with a 'normal' comfortable working distance.

Users may be able to use CCTV for a longer duration of time than optical devices.

The major disadvantages of a CCTV include:

They are bulky

They are more expensive than other low vision devices

They require a longer period of training compared to optical devices, for the patient to use them efficiently.

Most require electricity, therefore can only be used when there is electricity.

Video Magnifiers

These are portable readers consisting of a portable control unit with a video camera which can be connected to a television unit. The Keeler Max video magnification system consists of a hand held-magnifier and a miniature video camera. The magnifier is used to scan the text to be read while the video camera sends an enlarged black and white image to the television screen. A small view button on the magnifier allows the user to switch the image from soft-image pictures and photographs to a high contrast mode for text legibility. There is also a negative high contrast (contrast reversal) facility which provides white letters on a black background for those who are light sensitive.

Some video magnifiers have a separate movable camera which is moved over the reading material by the patient to project the image on the screen. The separate camera can also be mounted on a stand, so that the printed material can be moved horizontally to scan the print. They may be connected to a home television screen too. The Eezee reader shown **Figure 8.18** below has a small fixed focus camera and a hand-held scanner. The scanner has two rollers in its base which allow smooth horizontal movement across the reading material. Polarity reversal is shown in An Ash Tech. TVi hand-held video magnifier (white print on black background).

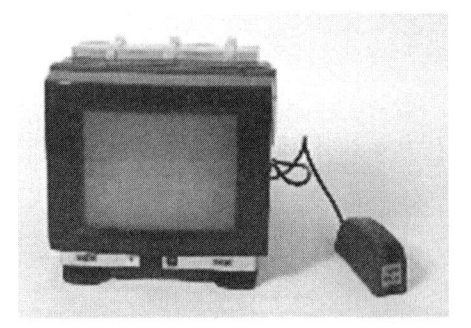

Figure 8.18: An Eezee Reader, consisting of a small hand-held camera connected to a screen monitor. Usually black on white, but may have reverse contrast (white on black) facility.

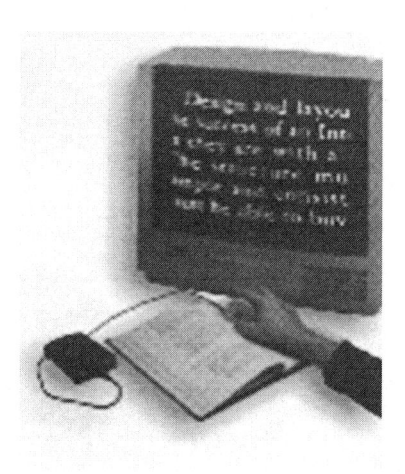

Figure 8.19: An Ash Tech. TVi hand-held video magnifier with reversed polarity (in negative photo selector, white print on black background). (Permission by Neville Clarence Technologies, NCTec).

The TVi (Figure 8.19) is a light, compact and portable electronic magnifier, ideal for use at home or in the classroom. Two models are currently available: the monochrome TVi classic with fixed magnification and the colour TVi with variable magnification. Both comprise of a mouse-type camera with in-built surface rollers and LED illumination, a compact control box and cable to connect to a standard PAL television which has an AV input. It can produce magnification from 22x to 43x on a large monitor such as 66 cm television monitor. Lower magnifications will be produced on smaller television screen monitors.

Ash Tech Prisma

One of the products of Ash Technology is the Prisma, a compact portable colour electronic magnifier which is ideal for home, school and office use. It consists of a camera mounted on a stand above a fixed reading platform (not X/Y sliding table). It has a large focus control, one-touch auto exposure. It produces a sharp, high contrast image and has a negative, positive and colour selector. A set includes a cable for connection to any standard PAL TV which has and AV input. The image can also be displayed on a personal computer or a laptop screen. It can offer magnification from 10x to 70x on a 66cm television screen. Lower magnifications will be produced on smaller television screen monitors.

Magnification provided by CCTV and video magnifiers

The magnification that may be provided on a screen depends on the type of the video magnifier. The magnification provided by this medium has been referred to as real image or transverse magnification. The prints are enlarged by a camera which is directly or indirectly linked to the screen. The size of the screen required is dependent on the degree of magnification desired. For high magnification, a large screen is desired, vice versa. Where patient's field limitation does not permit very high magnification, a small screen may be necessary. The magnification of a video magnifier consists of relative size magnification (RSM) and relative distance magnification (RDM)[4]. Therefore, total magnification M_{total} provided is $M_{rel\ size} \times M_{rel\ dist}$.

Relative size (basic) magnification is a measure of the size of the print or object on the screen. This magnification may reduce the field of vision and may be varied by varying the size of the monitor and / or the accessory lens system. The relative distance component is provided by the proximity (moving closer) to the screen. The visual field afforded by the device is not reduced by RSM magnification. Relative size magnification involving magnification of objects such as letters, and relative distance magnification (approach magnification) involving reduction viewing distance methods are common devices used to improve vision[4.] found these methods to be more commonly used among low vision patients.

An example of the total magnification provided by a video magnifier can be explained as follows:

If the basic magnification provided by the magnifier is 10x

If the viewing distance is 40 cm (requiring +2.50 D add or accommodation).

The total magnification is 10 X 2.50 = 25x.

If the viewing distance is reduced to 25 cm (requiring +4.00D add or accommodation).

The total magnification is 10 X 4 = 40x.

The viewing distance in each case is obviously more than that of an optical system that will provide similar magnifications.

For low vision patients with fast reading speeds, the minimum magnification for maximum visual field size would be advised. For patients who read slowly, the reading speed may improve at a higher magnification despite the reduced visual field size.

Video Magnifiers Interfaced with Personal Computer Systems

With the facility for interfacing video magnifiers with computer systems and television screens, more people with low vision are able to use video magnifiers. Computer video magnifiers (Video Graphic Array monitors) provide enlarged image of the print on the screen. Low vision patients can access personal computer in large prints as any personal computers can provide enlarged prints size which can be read by many low vision patients. There are many types of commercially available computer workstations for the low vision patient. Also, there are several computer adaptation magnifying systems consisting of a computer control unit and a camera unit (**Figure 8.20**) which permit printed or handwritten material to be read in enlarged form on the screen. The camera is placed on the reading material and an appropriate magnification selected.

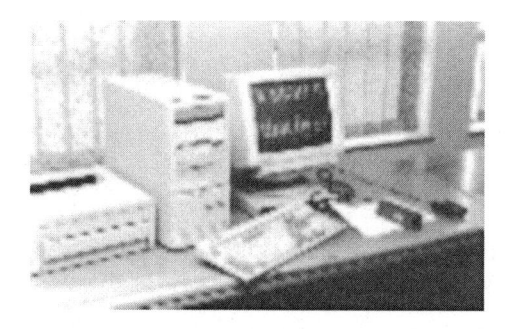

Figure 8.20: A hand held video camera unit attached to a personal computer system.

The camera is subsequently rolled over the material to be read to produce an enlarged image of the print on the screen. They can provide magnification of up to 32x. The advantage of such print is that they have a high contrast and the larger the screen of the computer, the larger the field of view, hence the larger the print that can be produced. Some systems afford image contrast in the form positive or negative image polarity. Some of these systems may permit writing or the completion of forms or writing cheques by the use of handwriting stands which can be used with the system. Placing the camera on the stand permits the magnification of the pen and paper to make it possible for the patient to write or complete forms. Some systems allow only a few words to be displayed at a time, while others may permit paragraphs to be displayed.

Head-Mounted Video Devices

Head-mounted video magnifiers have the advantages of CCTV with the portability of optical magnifiers. The low vision enhancement system consists of a headset containing a binocular, battery-powered, black-and-white video display that is attached to a control box. It is equipped with two video cameras having fixed focus magnification optics for orientation, and a centre-mounted camera with variable focus, and variable magnification optics for near, intermediate and distance tasks. It also incorporates a user-controlled electronic contrast enhancement feature, and an automatic compensation of camera sensitivity for changing light levels. The developers of the system recommend that they can be used for reading, writing, and other activities such as knitting and watching television[5]. They are, however, not recommended for walking because of the reduced field with increasing magnification which adversely affects mobility[6]. The advantages include the provision of high magnification, contrast enhancement and binocular viewing, while the high cost is a major disadvantage.

Text-to-speech conversion

Severely visually disabled and blind patients can also be assisted by Electronic technology as there are computer programmes which allow the low vision patient to use the keyboard to navigate the computer while texts are converted to speech using the computer's multimedia resources or an eternal device called speech synthesizer. Printed materials can be scanned into the computer as well and converted to Braille print. This permits the low vision patient who can read Braille to read non-visually. This can also be accessed via the speech synthesizer. Information can also be scanned onto the computer, and this can be magnified on the computer screen.

Environmental Modifications

Environmental modifications such as increasing or reducing illumination in a room or a child who needs more illumination to see better to sit close to the window, or a child who is photophobic, to sit away from the window, are common non-optical device (methods) of helping low vision patients. Appropriate signage for the low vision students around the school environment are essential. Also, it is essential that the room and compound where a visually impaired person lives must be well organized. Environmental assessment and modification have been found to be effective way of preventing falls among visually impaired elderly[7].

References

1. Rosenblum YZ, Zak PP, Ostrovsky MA, Smolyaninova IL, Bora EV, Dyadina UV Trofimova NN, Aliyev AGD. Spectral filters in low-vision correction. <u>Ophthal Physiol Optics</u>. 2000; 20: 335-341.

2. Cedrun-Sanchez, JE, Chamorro E, Bonnin-arias C, Aguirre-Vilacoro V, Castro Jj, Sachez-Ramos C. (2016)Visual discrimination increase by yellow filters in retinitis pigmentosa. Optom Vis Sci. 93; 12: 1537-1544.

3. Dickinson C. Low vision assessment - part two. Optician. 1993; 206: 25-31.

4. Lovie-Kitchin IL, and Woo GC. Effect of magnification and field of view on reading speed using a CCTV. Ophthal Pysiol opt. 1988; 8: 139-145.

5. Ortiz A, Chung ST, Legge GE and Jobling JT. Reading with a head-mounted video magnifier. Optom Vis Sci. 1999 76 755-762.

Bibliography

Eperjesi F, Fowler, CW, Evans BJ. Effects of filters on reading speed in normal and low vision due to age-related macular degeneration. Ophthal. Physiol Optics. 2004; xxx 17-25.

Hill S, Write M. Lighting for low vision: The office environment. Optician. 1999; 217: 28-32.

La Grow SJ, Roberston MC, Kerse MM. Reducing hazard related falls in people 75 years and older with significant visual impairment: how did a successful program work? Inj. Prev. 2006; 12: 296-301.

Massof RW and Richman DL. Obstacles encountered in the development of the low vision enhancement system. Optom Vis Sci 1992; 69: 32-41.

Monteiro MMB, Montilha RCI, Carvalho KMM, Gasparetto MERF. Optical and non-optical aids for reading and writing in individuals with acquired low vision. Arg. Bras. Oftalmol. 2014; 77:

Zabel L, Bouma H, and Mellote HE. Use of the TV magnifier in the Netherlands: A survey. J Vis Impair Blind. 1982; 76: 25-28.

Chapter 9
Visual Field Enhancement for Low Vision Patients

Apart from reduced visual acuity, loss of visual field is a common cause of low vision. There are many eye diseases that may result in visual filed loss, and the degree of disability varies from one disease to the other. Also, while a genetic condition such as juvenile macular degeneration may affect the central vision, resulting in serious central visual acuity loss, *retinitis pigmentosa*, also a genetic condition may cause peripheral visual filed loss, eventually leading to tunnel vision. Persons with central or peripheral visual field loss face significant environmental, social and perhaps, psychological problems.

While the major consequence of central visual filed loss is reading disability, the major impact of peripheral field loss relates to environmental navigation, bumping into objects, risk of fall and injury. Those with central field loss can be assisted with various forms of magnification, those with severe peripheral field loss cannot be helped by any form of magnification, but instead, they may benefit from minification. There are several devices for expanding visual field for the benefit of the patients with peripheral visual field loss.

Several methods of minification can be employed to enhance the visual field so that a significant part of the object or objects desired to be viewed, can be accommodated in the residual visual field of the patient. Also, depending on the type of field loss, patients can benefit significantly from mirror or prisms treatment. These will help to re-orientate the residual field of vision. The prism method is more common and provides better cosmesis.

Helping Patients with Peripheral Field Loss (restricted field)
Minifiers (Negative Lens Field Expander)

Conditions such as retinal degeneration resulting from *retinitis pigmentosa* or Usher's syndrome can cause a progressive loss of peripheral visual field, the advanced stage of which is referred to as tunnel vision and creates a lot of difficulty for the patient in navigating the environment. Patients with peripheral visual field loss may be rehabilitated. To assist patients with such severe peripheral field loss to increase their field hence improve their orientation and mobility in a strange environment, a minifier or field expansion device (Figure 9.1) may be used. This is a hand-held large diameter negative lens to be placed at a specific distance in front of the eye[1]. This is the simplest method of enhancing reduced peripheral visual field.

The concept of field expansion with negative lens field expander simply means that the patient will be able to see more objects in the field, however, the objects may appear small in size. A negative lens field expander is analogous to a reverse Galilean telescope, which minifies an object of regard. The hand-held negative lens represents the object lens of the reverse telescope and the accommodation of the patient represents the ocular lens (eyepiece). Where patient has insufficient accommodation, a positive Fresnel lens may be attached to the patient's standard spectacle, in which case the lens represents the ocular lens of the reverse telescope[2].

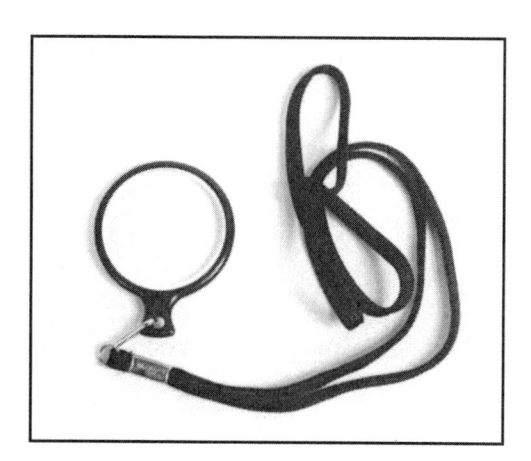

Figure 9.1: A negative lens field expander (minifier)

The location of the lens in front of the eye is critical. The maximum distance, t at which a lens of diameter d should be held from the eye's nodal point can be calculated by the formula: $t = d/ 2 \tan \theta$ (Kozlowski et al., 1984)[2]. Where t is the lens distance from the nodal point of the eye, d is the diameter of the lens (meters), and θ is half of the angle of the patient's remaining visual field. If angle θ is small and in radians, $\tan \theta = \theta$, therefore $t = d/2\theta$. However, if the angle is in degrees, the value of $t = 30 \, d/ \theta$, as 60 radians make one degree. The calculated magnification value using this device will be less than one, implying minification, which is necessary to expand the visual field.

Visual Field Expansion with Inverted Telescopes

An inverted telescope can also assist patients with peripheral field loss to expand their visual field. This minifies the object and the environment, thereby providing a greater field of view for the patient. A bioptic form of a peripheral vision-enhancement lens can help in these cases. The amorphic lenses have been designed to increase the peripheral vision field by minifying the horizontal meridian. The patient spends the majority of the time viewing through a carrier lens while the amorphic lens would be used transiently to spot and localize peripheral field information. The amorphic lenses are available in minifying powers ranging from –0.2 to –2.00 in increment of 0.2) and are to be prescribed, based on the highest power that the patient is comfortable with while walking[3].

The patient's distance prescription is to be incorporated into the carrier lenses and into the amorpic lenses. The location in which the lenses are to be mounted will depend on the patient's comfort, and frequent head movements. In addition, they may be mounted inferiorly on the carrier lenses. This system requires that the patient should be provided with an extensive training for effective use. A major disadvantage of this device is that it may be more expensive than the negative lens expander.

Visual Field Expansion with Prisms

Reduced visual field with relatively good visual acuity is an asset because, the possibility that assistance can be received in terms of optometric rehabilitation process is high. Patients with 10° to 15° of visual field and visual acuity of 6/30 (20/100) (0.7 logMAR) or better, will benefit from prism treatment. Even patients with 5° visual field or less with no peripheral island of vision may be good candidates, if they have adopted a fixed pattern of gaze[4]. As a rule, in the use of a prism to enhance visual field, the base of the prism is always towards the field loss area, so that the apex of the prism may bring the image from the non-seeing area to the seeing area of the field.

For a patient with binocular peripheral field loss, for each eye, base-in prism is applied nasally and a base-out prism is applied temporally to a carrier lens to bring peripheral objects into the field of vision[4]. A major disadvantage of prism management is the need for extensive training before the patient can adjust to the use of prism for mobility needs. Patients with visual field loss will benefit from this type of prism treatment, if given good training in mobility and scanning techniques[5]. Prism application may be achieved by using Weiss technique as follows:

- The patient wears his or her distance correction lenses in a carrier spectacle.
- With the patient's head in primary position of gaze, one eye occluded, the patient is instructed to fixate a distance object such as an acuity letter in about 2 lines above the best visual acuity in that eye.
- Precut paper strips of increasing widths are stuck vertically in front of the spectacle lens of the fixating eye until the residual temporal and nasal fields are just reached.
- Without changing the head or gaze position, the procedure is repeated for the other eye
- The strips are carefully taped to the front of the spectacle carrier lens over each eye.
- To ensure accuracy of the strip positions, the patient is instructed to look to the right and then to the left binocularly without moving the head, to recheck the position of the strips.
- It is important that both eyes see simultaneously with the strips on.
- A 15^Δ base-out Fresnel prism membrane is then applied to the back of the carrier lens, 1 millimetre external to the edge of the temporal paper strip.
- A 15^Δ base-in Fresnel prism membrane is also applied to the back of the lens, 1 millimetre internal to the edge of the nasal paper strip, parallel to the base of the first membrane

Other than the 15^Δ stated above, other values such as 20^Δ or even 30^Δ have been proposed. Also, it is recommended that the temporal field be fitted first, and after the patient has adjusted to this, the nasal field should be fitted[5]. Since the inferior field is important for the mobility of the patient, it has been suggested that base-down prisms may be added below the horizontal ones to increase the inferior vertical field. It is important to note that prisms are not comfortable for constant wear due to disorientation[1].

Homonymous Hemianopia

Homonymous hemianopia (or homonymous hemianopsia) is hemianopic visual field loss on the same side of both eyes, which may be on the right side, left side, up or down. Prisms can be applied to enhance visual field in the areas of loss. The vertical edge of a Fresnel prism is applied to each lens with the base directed towards the affected field. For the nasal field loss, the prism is placed base-in, and for the temporal field loss, the prism base out. The prism should be applied in such a way that its apex is 2 millimetres from the edge of the pupil to avoid interference with the central vision[5].

Management of patients with visual field loss require sincere patience and commitment, because some of the processes involved, especially the training in the use of the devices may be frustrating, both to the practitioner and the patient. However, both of them will be happy with the successful provision of useful expanded visual fields.

References

Woo GC. Ing B, Lee M. Determining the power of a negative lens expander. Clin Exp Optom. 2001; 84:162-164.

Kozlowski JM, Mainster MA and Avila MP. Negative lens field expander. Arch Ophthalmol. 1984; 102: 1182-1184.

Szlyk JP, Seiple W, Laderman DJ, Kelsch R, Ho K, Mcmahon T. Use of bioptic amorphic lenses to expand the visual field in patients with peripheral field loss. Optom Vis Sci. 1998; 75: 518-524.

Veronneau-Troutman S. Prisms in the medical and surgical management of strabismus. St. Louis, Mosby 1994. 59.

Feraro J. Jose R, Olssen L. Frenel prism as a treatment option for retinitis pigmentosa. Tex Optom. 1982; 38: 18-20.

D. a two-stage hypothesis for the neural cause of retinitis pigmentosa. Adv Biosci. 1987; 62: 29-58.

Mehlata M. An RP patient's description of her visual disturbance. Advances in Biosciences. 1987; 63: 175-180.

Nilsson UL. Visual rehabilitation of patients with advanced stages of glaucoma, myopia or retinitis pigmentosa. Doc. Ophthalmol. 1998; 70: 363-383.

Chapter 10
Incorporating Low Vision Care Into an Eye Care Practice

As stated in chapter one, low vision (partial sight) in the context of this book, refers to visual acuity worse than 6/18 but better than 3/60 in the better eye, that cannot be corrected by medical or surgical intervention and or refractive error correction. Low vision also refers to visual field less than 20 degrees but better than 10 degrees in the better eye. These definitions imply that anyone who has low vision cannot be assisted by conventional eye care. Visual impairment is globally prevalent in both adults and children and according to the World Health Organization (WHO, 2002), there were more than 161 million visually impaired people. Thirty-seven millions of these were blind and 124 million had low vision. Therefore, low vision is one of the major health problems world-wide.

Low vision has significant impact on performance of daily living activities, and consequently, on the quality of life of those with the condition. However, low vision patients can be assisted to perform certain limited desired tasks by vision rehabilitation, encapsulated in low vision care. As shown in chapter three of this book, comprehensive approach to low vision is the recommended method to enhance visual improvement, hence quality of life (QoL) for individuals with the condition.

Unfortunately, low vision care services are scanty in many countries of the world, especially in the developing countries. This is surprising, as low vision care is one of the specialty areas in Optometry curricula in many countries. Low vision rehabilitation is part of eye care services that optometrists should offer to their patients. Worldwide, however, not many eye care practitioners (optometrist and ophthalmologists) engage in this aspect of eye care, and the reasons for this may include the following:

Lack of interest in low vision care

Lack of appropriate knowledge needed for the practice

Low vision care is time-consuming

Economic reasons, low vision is not lucrative

Stereotypical perception that most low vision patients do not benefit from this service

Lack of knowledge on how low vision care may be incorporated into the general optometric practice.

The purpose of this chapter, is to encourage eye care practitioners to incorporate low vision services into their practices and suggest how this could be done. This will be an important step towards increasing the number of centres where low vision services can be accessed. With such incorporation, interest will be generated, skill will be developed. Interestingly, many present facilities where eye care services are located can accommodate low vision care. Also, many of the equipment that are currently used to examine patients, are part of those needed for low vision care. Further, most basic trial low vision devices needed to examine low vision patients are inexpensive, hence affordable. Furthermore, a few, for example, spectacle and, hand-held magnifiers are easily accessible from local optical suppliers. Spectacle magnifiers, typoscopes and a few other devices can be made by the practitioner. If available, a separate consulting room may be dedicated to low vision care, and a day should be set aside for that service, and arrangement made for patients to be booked for that day.

The following need to be known by practitioners, regarding incorporation of low vision care into an existing eye care practice:

Basic knowledge of low vision patient assessment

Knowledge of calculation of magnification required by the patient

Basic diagnostic equipment and devices (optical and non-optical) needed for low vision patient assessment

Possible referral sources for low vision patients

Professional colleagues to whom patients may be referred

Operative knowledge on assessment and prescribing devices for low vision patients.

Need for mentorship by existing low vision practitioner

Need for continuing education via conferences journals and books.

Basic Knowledge Of Low Vision Patient Assessment

In order to incorporate low vision care into eye care practice, it is important for the practitioner to refresh his or her knowledge of low vision patient assessment, which can be found in any standard low vision textbook, including Chapters 4 and 5 of this book. The procedures are generally similar to those of the assessment of normally sighted patients, although there are few differences, and these are highlighted in chapters on assessments of adult and children with low vision.

Knowledge of Calculation of Magnification Required by the Patient

There are several methods of calculating magnification needed by low vision patients, some are simple, and others are complex. A few of the simple ones are briefly described in Chapter 7. Anyone wishing to incorporate low vision into his or her practice is advised to be conversant with at least one or two methods of calculating magnifications in view of prescribing devices for low vision patients.

Basic Diagnostic Equipment

Many of the basic equipment for examining low vision patients are mostly the same as those that are used to examine normally sighted patients in any eye care practice, and are listed below:

Diagnostic instrument {Retinoscope and ophthalmoscope (direct and or indirect)} and pen torch

Trial lens box, preferably full aperture lenses with usual accessories, and appropriate trial frames for children and adults.

Hand-held Jackson cross cylinders (± 1.0 and ± 2.0)

Low vision visual acuity charts (various types for distance and near). Examples: Feinbloom distance acuity test chart, Bailey and Lovie distance chart. For near: Lighthouse near acuity test, LogMAR near alphabet and continuous charts for low vision.

Contrast sensitivity charts (e.g. Vistech or Peli-Robson chart)

Slit lamp

Tonometer (e.g. Schiotz)

Colour vision test (e.g. Farnsworth Panel D-15 which is easy to administer and score)

Visual field testing equipment {e.g. Tangent (Bjerrum) screen for distance and Amsler grid for near}.

Others such as acuity chart for low vision patients can be purchased.

Basic Low Vision Optical Devices

Basic optical devices include spectacle, hand-held, and stand magnifiers, and telescopes. A few of these could be purchased initially to commence low vision care services. Others such as Electronic devices can be purchased as the low vision care services expand. The following power (magnifications) are recommended.

Spectacle magnifiers: +6.00 (1.5x) +8.00 (2x), +10.00 (2.5x) and +12.00D (3x) (half eye and full eye with prisms).

Hand magnifiers: 1.5x, 2x, 3x, 3.5x, 4x, 6x or higher

Stand magnifiers: Dome magnifier (1.5x, 2x and 3x) standard stand magnifiers (2x, 3x, 4x) bar magnifier e.g. ruler type (1.5, 2x), suspended chest magnifier (2x)

Telescopes: Monocular/binocular: e.g. distance (2x, 2.5, 3x) and near (2.5, 3x, 4x).

These various devices and others are discussed in chapter 8.***Basic low vision non-optical devices***

Sunshades: should be dark enough to reduce glare, but not too dark to reduce vision e.g. grey, amber, brown, green.

Typoscopes (can be self-made)

Others that can be prescribed for the patient to buy: visors, hats with wide brim, umbrellas (for those who are disturbed by sunlight).

These and other non-optical devices are discussed in Chapter 9.

Electronic devices: Closed circuit television (CCTV), computer programmes as discussed in chapter 9, could be acquired later as the services expand.

Low Vision Patient Referral Sources

It is important for the low vision practitioner to know what his or her referral sources are. Common referral sources, depending on the location of the practice, would include the following:

Other optometrists

Ophthalmologists

Schools for the blind, the disabled etc.
Society for the blind
Old age homes
Psychologists or psychiatrists
Social workers
Occupational therapists
Hospitals
Existing patients

The practitioner must introduce himself to the above professionals and establishments.

Referral from the Low Vision Practitioner

The professionals to whom the low vision care practitioner may refer patients to, depending on the need of each patient, include the following:

- Ophthalmologists
- Psychologists or psychiatrists
- Social workers
- Occupational therapists.
- Special educators

Other possible service providers that the low vision practitioner may wish to refer patients to, depending on the need of the patient, are discussed in chapter 3. When a patient is being referred, a referral letter should be provided for him or her narrating the chief complaint of the patient and other concerns, tests that have been conducted, findings including diagnoses, why the patient is being referred, and what assistance is expected from the professional.

Operative Knowledge

In addition to the information provided above, which are very pertinent to low vision practice, the following operative knowledge need to be acquired by the practitioner.

Basic low vision patient assessment procedure.
Calculation of magnifier powers.
Knowledge of appropriate devices and where they can be purchased
Education and training procedures for the devices.

Knowledge of cost of devices is essential for communication to the patient

Knowledge of sources of financial support for the patient is essential because of patient who might need devices but unable to afford them

Mentorship and Continuing Education

The new practitioner will benefit from the mentorship of existing practitioners in the field. He or she should liaise with such practitioner, so that when necessary, the existing practitioner can be consulted for his or her views on a case, or any issue that is not clear to him or her. Practitioners are encouraged to engage in continuing education programme by attending conferences and seminars on low vision care, reading journal articles and textbooks on low vision care, and other relevant materials.

Bibliography

Bailey IL. Refracting low vision patients. Optom monthly. 1978; 69: 131-134.

Birch J. Color deficiency: An introduction. Optician. 1999; 218: 22-25.

Brower J. A practical guide to low vision assessment and dispensing. Optom today. 2001; Feb. 9: 34-36.

Dijk KV. Low vision care: who can help? Comm. Eye Health J. 2012; 25: 14-15.

Eperjesi F, Fowler CW, Evans BJ. Effects of filters on reading speed in normal and low vision due to age-related macular degeneration. Ophthal Physiol Optics. 2004; 24: 17-25.

Fortney GL, Krohn MA. The limitations of kinetic perimetry in early scotoma detection. Ophthalmol. 1978; 85: 287-293.

Leat S, Rumney N. A simplified approach to low vision assessment. 1. Optician 1990; Sep 14: 11-19.

Lovie-Kitchin JE, Whittaker SG. Prescribing near magnification for low vision patients. Clin Exp Optom. 1999; 82: 214-224.

Minto H. Establishing low vision services at secondary level. Com Eye Heath J. 2004; 17: 5-7.

Monteiro MMB, Montilha RCI, Carvalho KMM, Gasparetto MERF. Optical and non-optical aids for reading and writing in individuals with acquired low vision. Arg. Bras. Oftalmol. 2014; 77: xxxx

Oduntan AO. Introducing low vision care into the Government eye care services in South Africa. S Afr Optom. 2007; 66: 163-175.

Runstrom MM, Eperjesi F. Is there a need for binocular vision evaluation in low vision? Opththal Physiol Optics. 1995; 15: 525-528.

Vision 2020 Low Vision Group. Standard list of low vision services. Comm Eye Health J. 2004: 17, (49) 5-8.

World Health Organization (WHO) 2009. Magnitude and causes of visual impairment. Available at http://www.who.int/mediacentre/factsheets/fs282/en/index.hotmail. Accessed May, 2002.

Professor Oduntan obtained B.Sc. (First Class Hons) from the Department of Optometry, University of Benin, Nigeria in 1982 and PhD, Optometry from the City University, London., UK, 1989. He was a Commonwealth Scholar. He was appointed Assistant Professor at the King Saud University, Saudi Arabia, (1989-1996), Associate Professor, University of Limpopo (UL), South Africa, (1996-2001) Professor, University of Limpopo (UL), South Africa, (2002-2008), Professor, University of KwaZulu-Natal, South Africa, (2008-2013) and Honorary Professor, University of KwaZulu-Natal, South Africa (2014 -2016). His research interest include Ocular anatomy, Design of eye care test charts, Eye Health Promotion and low vision care. He has published over 70 research articles in peer-reviewed journals. Major research achievements include discovery of an elastic tissue layer in the primate conjunctiva (J. Anat. 1989, 163: 165-172); Description of the source of sensory innervation of the inferior conjunctiva (Graefe's Arch. Ophthalmol.1992, 230:258-263), Description of organization of capillaries in the primate conjunctiva. (Ophthalmic Res. 1992, 40-44) and report on the causes and prevalence of low vision and blindness in the Limpopo Province of South Africa. S. Afr Optom. 2003, 62: 8-15. He is the author of a monograph: Global visual impairment: Epidemiology, implications and prevention. University of Limpopo Press, 2005, (ISBN 0-9584778-8-4) and a chapter in a book: The role of psychotherapy in the contemporary rehabilitation of visually impaired patients. In: Madu NS (editor). Mental health and Psychology in Africa. World Council for Psychotherapy, African Chapter, UL Publisher, Polokwane, 2005 and completed a book manuscript: Contemporary low vision care. He has supervised several Master and PhD students. Professor Oduntan joined the Department of Optometry, Madonna University, Elele, Rivers States, Nigeria in April 2014.